Palliative Care

SECOND EDITION

Christina Faull

Consultant in Palliative Medicine, LOROS, The Leicestershire
and Rutland Hospice and the University Hospitals of Leicester

Honorary Professor of Palliative Medicine, Centre for
Promotion of Excellence in Palliative Care, de Montfort
University, Leicester

and

Kerry Blankley

Education Facilitator, LOROS, The Leicestershire and Rutland
Hospice

Honorary Lecturer, Centre for Promotion of Excellence in
Palliative Care, de Montfort University, Leicester

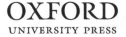

OXFORD
UNIVERSITY PRESS

OXFORD
UNIVERSITY PRESS

Great Clarendon Street, Oxford, OX2 6DP,
United Kingdom

Oxford University Press is a department of the University of Oxford.
It furthers the University's objective of excellence in research, scholarship,
and education by publishing worldwide. Oxford is a registered trade mark of
Oxford University Press in the UK and in certain other countries

First Edition published in 2002
Second Edition published in 2015

Impression: 1

Published in the United States of America by Oxford University Press
198 Madison Avenue, New York, NY 10016, United States of America

British Library Cataloguing in Publication Data
Data available

Library of Congress Control Number: 2014958221

ISBN 978-0-19-870241-2

Printed in Great Britain by
Clays Ltd, St Ives plc

Preface

All doctors and nurses need to know how best to care for patients with advanced, life- limiting disease and those who are dying. This is true also for many other professionals who support patients in their homes, in care homes, and in hospital. Patients need us to be knowledgeable, skilful, and understanding. This book outlines the fundamental principles and facts which will enable you to make a very real difference to your patients and their families. In addition, it has been found that by increasing your confidence in providing such care, you will gain greater professional satisfaction.

The care of patients with advanced and terminal illness can be extremely rewarding but often causes professionals a considerable amount of discomfort. This is especially so when they feel under-confident in their abilities to provide a high quality of symptom management and relief from distress and to communicate appropriately with patients. Patients with advanced disease present some of the most challenging ethical, physical, psychological, and social issues to clinicians and, indeed, to society. Their care requires a true integration of the art and science of medicine. The last part of life is filled with loss, celebration, re-evaluation, regrets, love, suffering, resolution, turmoil, and peace. It is small wonder that their care is sometimes uncomfortable!

Since the first edition of this book, thirteen years ago, the emphasis on the provision of high-quality palliative and end of life care has increased, and palliative care methods are now seen as important, effective, and central to routine clinical practice, both in hospital and the community. The curricula for many professional groups has been developed and this book draws on many of them, in particular, the common core competences for end of life care (Chapter 8). Knowing what you need to know is important; you want to be efficient in your learning. To help you, we have included this curriculum in questionnaire form so that you can assess your own strengths and weaknesses and make an action plan for your learning. Competency is required in:

◆ communication

◆ amelioration of suffering, the relief of pain and other symptoms

◆ assessment and care planning

◆ anticipatory planning, with patients and their families, for times of deterioration.

It is also vital to develop attitudes which enable professionals to work most effectively and sensitively with people with incurable illness, who are facing the certainty of death, within their own psychosocial and cultural context.

This book aims to be both a practical resource and to provoke contemplative professional development. Whilst focused primarily at nursing and medical students and newly registered, it will be of use to students in other clinical disciplines and professional groups. We know that we all learn in different ways. Some are very good at reading text and remembering; others prefer to learn more by experience. This book aims to appeal to a broad range of learning styles by presenting information in different ways. Hopefully, the variety will make it interesting and enjoyable, therefore enhancing your learning.

We hope, by the end of this book, you feel better prepared to help patients and families at a time of great need.

C. F. and K.B.
2015

Acknowledgements

This book could not have been completed without the support of our partners, Jon and Andrew, and their generosity in creating the time for us to write.

We should also like to acknowledge the wonderful work of Dr Richard Woof on the first edition of this book and the help of Chris Birtwistle and Brigitte Jones for this second edition.

Contents

Palliative care: principles, challenges, and patient outcomes

Chapter 1

Palliative care: principles, challenges, and patient outcomes

Your dying patient needs you

It seems still to be the case that, in practice, the discussion of death as an inevitable and, in some cases, imminent aspect of life is regarded as morbid and thus avoided. Even with patients suffering from terminal conditions, it is common for there to have been no discussion with patients, their consultants or GPs, relatives, and carers, about preparing for dying.[1]

Review of the Liverpool Care Pathway, 2013, reproduced under the Open Government Licence v.2.0

On my very first day of working in a hospital I was faced with the care of a 56-year-old man, waking up from a temazepam overdose which he had taken because of his incurable lung cancer. He didn't want to face the future likelihood of pain, loss of independence, and loss of dignity. He felt useless. He was deeply regretful; both for the hurt he had caused his family and of the fact that he had failed to kill himself. He was withdrawn and chose to lie in bed with his eyes tightly closed. I felt ill-equipped to help this man and his family. I muddled through. I remember it as scary. One of those patients I'll never forget. This man and the problems he had didn't fit into the model I had of health care. Taking his 'history' revealed the physical symptoms of the lung cancer. It all appeared miserable. I felt helpless and struggled with my agreement with his reasons for wanting to die. I wanted to do something to make things better but I couldn't do anything about the cancer.

As a doctor, nurse, or allied health professional you will often be caring for people with incurable fatal conditions, managing the problems of advanced diseases, looking after patients who are dying, and supporting their families. This presents a challenge unlike any other, most especially when you are newly qualified and lacking experience, knowledge, and skills. Looking after people who are going to die soon is often both sad and difficult. It is also very rewarding and can sometimes bring great joy and even fun. Figure 1.1 captures some of the thoughts that may arise in this area of patient care.

None of us wants to 'muddle through' and fail to help patients when they need help most. The specialty of palliative care has developed to guide us. Like any other

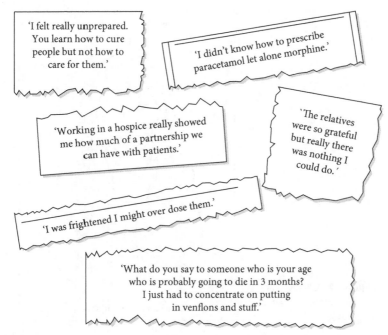

Figure 1.1 Some thoughts of newly qualified practitioners caring for patients with advanced illness

clinical discipline, there is an evidence base, recommended standards of good practice, and defined competences and curriculum for doctors, nurses and others in training (see Chapter 8). Whatever branch of health you eventually specialize in, you will be responsible for patients with palliative care needs and you will need to be confident that you can palliate their symptoms and reduce their distress.

Just because you can't cure them, doesn't mean you can't have a dramatic effect on their quality of life and the way they die. There is *always* something you can do. Palliative care should not be seen as an optional extra, for the patient or for you (Figure 1.2). It should be an integrated part of the way we all work as health care professionals.

You have the potential to really make a difference for patients. You can use your knowledge of drugs to alleviate suffering. You can speak with patients to understand what they want and help them get it. You really do have a great chance to help, usually much more than you think.

What is palliative care?

To help us understand how we can best help dying patients, the World Health Organization has agreed a definition and principles of palliative care.[2]

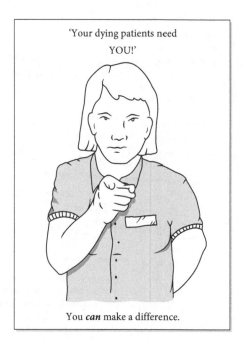

'Your dying patients need
YOU!'

You *can* make a difference.

Figure 1.2 Palliative care is not an optional extra for your patient

Box 1.1 The principles of palliative care (adapted from WHO definition)[2]

- Affirms life and regards dying as a normal process.
- Intends to neither hasten nor postpone death.
- Provides relief from pain and other distressing symptoms.
- Integrates the psychological, physical, social, and spiritual aspects of a patient's care (holism).
- Supports patients to live as actively as possible until death.
- Supports the family during the patient's illness and in their own bereavement.
- Uses a team approach to address the needs of patients and their families.
- Is applicable early in the course of illness, in conjunction with other therapies that are intended to prolong life.

Adapted with permission from World Health Organization, *National Cancer Control Programmes: Policies and Managerial Guidelines*, Second edition, World Health Organization, Geneva, Switzerland, Copyright © 2002.

Box 1.2 Definition of palliative care[2]

Palliative care is an approach that improves the quality of life of patients and their families facing the problems associated with life-threatening illness, through the prevention and relief of suffering by means of early identification and impeccable assessment and treatment of pain and other problems, physical, psychosocial and spiritual.

Reproduced with permission from World Health Organization, *National Cancer Control Programmes: Policies and Managerial Guidelines,* Second edition, World Health Organization, Geneva, Switzerland, Copyright © 2002.

The goals of palliative care are to achieve the best possible quality of life for patients and their families, to facilitate adjustment to the many losses they will face, and to attain a dignified death, with minimum distress, in the patient's place of choice. The principles of care that are used to achieve these goals are identified in Box 1.1 (see also Box 1.2). The picture and words created by Michele Petrone in Figure 1.3 capture how a patient with cancer expresses this need for palliative care.

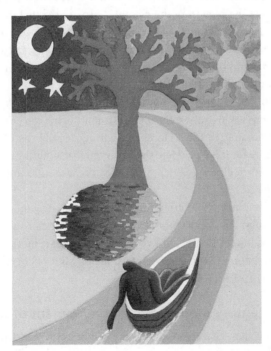

Figure 1.3 The journey to where?[3]

Image reproduced with permission of The Michele Angelo Petrone Foundation, <www.makingartpersonal.org>

I don't know where my life will take me. I don't know how the river bends or where
the rapids may be. Radiotherapy completed my treatment, but my journey isn't
finished. My cancer seems to be gone, but who can be sure? There are no
certainties, and from time to time a new pain has panicked myself and my loved
ones. My body may be healed now but adjusting to the changes in my life and the
recovery of my emotions, my soul, and my spirit takes longer.[3]

Poem reproduced with permission of The Michele Angelo Petrone Foundation,
<www.makingartpersonal.org>

A little bit of history

Perhaps it is that each era of history or each generation of doctors has its champions of the care of the dying. Hippocrates was, of course, a great orator on the subject, and in the Victorian era, when the medical profession in the United Kingdom was really beginning to shape itself, Sir Henry Halford (president of the Royal College of Physicians for 24 years) and William Munk (another key figure in the College) were leading proponents. Munk published an early palliative care textbook in 1887 entitled *Euthanasia: Or Medical Treatment in Aid of an Easy Death*.[4] In Munk's book, the term *euthanasia* was used in its literal Greek sense of *good death*. It has since become a term used when a life is intentionally ended at the request of the patient. Munk noted that medical schools didn't include teaching about how to care for patients who were dying and that young doctors often were unprepared for this when they started work on the wards. It wasn't until this century, however, that this became embedded in the curriculum for medical students.

Nursing and care of the dying may be seen as natural partners. The concepts of whole-person care, dignity, suffering, and quality of life can be found through the history of nursing. In 1859, Florence Nightingale published *Notes on Nursing: What It Is, What It Is Not*.[5] Here she observed that suffering extends beyond the bodily effects of illness and that nursing can relieve suffering without treating the disease.

In spite, indeed maybe because of the advent of the new therapeutics in the twentieth century, the importance of the role of the doctor in the care of the dying became a lower priority until very recently. What is more, doctors in the mid twentieth century became fearful of using opioids for pain relief because of the perceived risk of addiction.

Twentieth-century pioneers and development of services

In the 1960s, two new champions of the care of dying emerged. Cicely Saunders founded St Christopher's Hospice in London in 1967 and established that regular giving of morphine to patients with cancer pain achieved excellent control of pain for the vast majority of people with no risk of addiction whatsoever. Dame Cicely, first a nurse, then a social worker, and thirdly a doctor, also re-established a philosophy of medicine that had been in danger of disappearing—that patients, in all their aspects and dimensions, are the concern of the doctor, not the disease alone[6] (see Chapter 3).

Elizabeth Kubler-Ross, an American psychiatrist, opened our minds to understanding the experiences of people who live with the knowledge that they will be dying in the near future. Her models of loss are fundamental to the way we have learned to provide support to patients and families[7] (see Chapter 3). Psychiatrists in the United Kingdom, Colin Murray Parkes and John Hinton, have made an enormous contribution to the success of our work with patients and with bereaved families, and established how important care of the bereaved is in promoting physical and mental health.[8,9]

The development of palliative care services has also been driven by 'users'. In 1911, Douglas Macmillan watched his father die of cancer. His father's pain and suffering moved Douglas to found The Society for the Prevention and Relief of Cancer, now called Macmillan Cancer Support. When the Hampstead-based Marie Curie Hospital was transferred to the NHS in 1948, a group of committee members from the hospital decided to preserve the name of Marie Curie in a charity dedicated to alleviating suffering from cancer —and is today known as Marie Curie Cancer Care. An extensive nationwide survey was undertaken to help identify medical, nursing, and research needs in relation to cancer. The results formed the basis of the work of the charity.

In the United Kingdom, there are now:

- 223 hospice and adult palliative care in-patient units
- 3200 hospice and palliative care beds
- 291 home care services
- 129 'Hospice at Home' services
- 275 day care centres
- 346 hospital support services
- 43 children's hospice in-patient units with 338 hospice beds.

(Read more about what these services provide in Chapter 9.)

Recent history

In 1988, palliative medicine became a specialty recognized by the Royal College of Physicians, just like other specialties such as cardiology or neurology.

The National End of Life Care Strategy for England and Wales was launched in 2008[10] and, in 2010, the General Medical Council in the United Kingdom

---

Box 1.3 GMC expectations of clinical teams[12]

- Identification of patients approaching the end of life
- Provision of information on this matter
- Determination of preferences regarding life-sustaining treatment including cardiopulmonary resuscitation
- Documentation of the above in an unambiguous and accessible format

Reproduced from Bell, D., GMC guidelines on end of life care, *British Medical Journal*, Volume 340, Number 761, pp.1373–1374, Copyright © 2010, with permission from BMJ Publishing Group.

---

recommended that death should be an explicit discussion point when patients are likely to die within 12 months.[11] Box 1.3 identifies the mandated expectations in this guidance.[12]

Who needs palliative care?

Around 1% of the population of the United Kingdom die each year; 500,000 people died in England and Wales in 2012, 84% of whom were over 65 years old. Nearly 200,000 people who died were 85 years old or more and, by 2030, it is thought that 44% of people who die will be over 85 years old. It is also likely that the number of people dying will have increased by 17% by 2030.

We know that in the United Kingdom, although most people would ideally wish to die at home,

- around 53% of people die in hospital;
- 20% of hospital beds are, at any one time, used for the care of patients with advanced disease;
- one-third of patients with advanced illness will die within a week of their final admission, but 40% will be in hospital for longer than 1 month;
- most hospital resources are used for people who are in the last year of their lives.

You will see a lot of people in hospital and in the community who have advanced disease, some of whom you will be caring for when they die. We know that it is difficult for many health professionals to identify whether a patient may be at risk of deteriorating and dying, especially those patients that don't

Supportive and Palliative Care Indicators Tool (SPICT™)

NHS Lothian

The SPICT™ is a guide to identifying people at risk of deteriorating and dying. Assessment of unmet supportive and palliative care needs may be appropriate.

Look for two or more general indicators of deteriorating health.

- Performance status poor or deteriorating, with limited reversibility. (needs help with personal care, in bed or chair for 50% or more of the day).
- Two or more unplanned hospital admissions in the past 6 months.
- Weight loss (5 – 10%) over the past 3 – 6 months and/or body mass index < 20.
- Persistent, troublesome symptoms despite optimal treatment of any underlying condition(s).
- Lives in a nursing care home or NHS continuing care unit, or needs care to remain at home.
- Patient requests supportive and palliative care, or treatment withdrawal.

Look for any clinical indicators of advanced conditions

Cancer

Functional ability deteriorating due to progressive metastatic cancer.

Too frail for oncology treatment or treatment is for symptom control.

Dementia/ frailty

Unable to dress, walk or eat without help.

Choosing to eat and drink less; difficulty maintaining nutrition.

Urinary and faecal incontinence.

No longer able to communicate using verbal language; little social interaction.

Fractured femur; multiple falls.

Recurrent febrile episodes or infections; aspiration pneumonia.

Neurological disease

Progressive deterioration in physical and/or cognitive function despite optimal therapy.

Speech problems with increasing difficulty communicating and/or progressive dysphagia.

Recurrent aspiration pneumonia; breathless or respiratory failure.

Heart/ vascular disease

NYHA Class III/IV heart failure, or extensive, untreatable coronary artery disease with:

- breathlessness or chest pain at rest or on minimal exertion.

Severe, inoperable peripheral vascular disease.

Respiratory disease

Severe chronic lung disease with:

- breathlessness at rest or on minimal exertion between exacerbations.

Needs long term oxygen therapy.

Has needed ventilation for respiratory failure or ventilation is contraindicated.

Kidney disease

Stage 4 or 5 chronic kidney disease (eGFR < 30ml/min) with deteriorating health.

Kidney failure complicating other life limiting conditions or treatments.

Stopping dialysis.

Liver disease

Advanced cirrhosis with one or more complications in past year:

- diuretic resistant ascites
- hepatic encephalopathy
- hepatorenal syndrome
- bacterial peritonitis
- recurrent variceal bleeds

Liver transplant is contraindicated.

Supportive and palliative care planning

- Review current treatment and medication so the patient receives optimal care.
- Consider referral for specialist assessment if symptoms or needs are complex and difficult to manage.
- Agree current and future care goals/ plan with the patient and family.
- Plan ahead if the patient is at risk of loss of capacity.
- Handover: care plan, agreed levels of intervention, CPR status.
- Coordinate care (eg. with a primary care register).

SPICT™, November 2013

Figure 1.4 Supportive and Palliative Care Indicator tool (SPICT)[13]

Reproduced from Highet, G. et al., Development and evaluation of the Supportive and Palliative Care Indicators Tool (SPICT): A mixed-methods study, *BMJ Supportive and Palliative Care*, Online First Article, DOI:10.1136/bmjspcare-2013–000488, Copyright © 2014, with permission from BMJ Publishing Group.

have cancer. People may be considered to be approaching the end of their life when they:

◆ might die within the next 12 months because of deterioration from a serious chronic health problem, including frailty;

◆ they have a life-threatening acute event;

◆ they have a serious underlying condition that puts them at risk of sudden death.

Sometimes tools can be helpful in thinking about whether a patient is at risk of deteriorating and dying and identifying that they may have unmet supportive and palliative care needs and could benefit from a review of care goals and anticipatory care planning. An example is the Supportive and Palliative Care Indicator Tool (SPICT)[13] (Figure 1.4). The SPICT is a web-based tool shared by an online community of professionals. You can register, join this community, and make sure you access the most up-to-date version at <http://www.spict. org.uk>

Some patients, those with chronic progressive illness and frailty, can be identified as being in their last 6–12 months, whereas other patients have a sudden illness with little prior ill health. In each of these time frames (Figure 1.5), the key to being able to provide good care is in identifying what may be happening to patients, sharing that information sensitively, and offering patients and their families the opportunity to make decisions about future care and plan appropriately for anticipated changes.

THE END OF LIFE				THEY DYING PHASE
At risk of dying in 6 – 12 months, but may live for years	MONTHS 2 – 9 months	SHORT WEEKS 1 – 8 weeks	LAST DAYS 2 – 14 days	LAST HOURS 0 – 48 hours
DISEASE(S) RELENTLESS Progression is less reversible Treatment benefits are waning	CHANGE UNDERWAY Benefit of treatment less evident Harms of treatment less tolerable	RECOVERY LESS LIKELY The risk of death is rising	DYING BEGINS Deterioration is weekly/daily	ACTIVELY DYING The body is shutting down The person is letting go

Figure 1.5 Time frames in the dying process[1]

Reproduced from *Independent Review of the Liverpool Care pathway: More Care, Less Pathway*, Williams Lea, London, UK, © Crown Copyright 2013, licensed under the Open Government Licence v.2.0.

How to care well for the dying

What do patients and their carers need?

The 'case history exercise' will help you think about what patients might need and your role in their care.

 CASE HISTORY EXERCISE

Mrs Ada Jones is a 62-year-old lady who lives with John, to whom she has been married for 5 years. She was divorced from Fred 10 years ago. They had four children together. John has two children from his previous marriage. Ada and John have 14 grandchildren and two great-grandchildren. She works as a dinner lady at the local primary school and loves playing indoor bowls. She was diagnosed with motor neurone disease (MND) 6 months ago and is now unable to walk. She has asked her GP to visit today because she has found that she is coughing when swallowing drinks.

Whatever your own profession, you may be asked to care for a patient like Mrs Jones and need to develop skills to support her. Although the GP has an important role in this situation, so too do all care professionals. Think about the following and what your professional role is.

♦ What do you think might be on Mrs Jones's mind?

♦ What do you think Mrs Jones might want from her GP (and from you)?

♦ What do you think the GP will be wanting to think about with her?

(See our thoughts in 'Case history exercise: some thoughts on Mrs Jones' later in this chapter.)

First and foremost, patients want us to see them as people. We know that this is a really vital part of preserving their dignity. Look at the extract from the poem 'Kate', thought to be written by Phyllis McCormack when she was a nurse in training:

So open your eyes, nurse
Open and see,
Not a crabbit old woman,
Look closer – See Me[14]

Phyllis McCormack, *Crabbit Old Woman*, 1966. First published in
Searle, C. (ed), *Elders*, Reality Press, London, UK, 1973

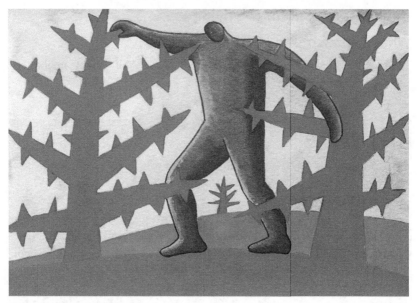

Figure 1.6 The pain of it all

Image reproduced with permission of The Michele Angelo Petrone Foundation, <www.makingartpersonal.org>

Perhaps a patient may be wanting to talk about dying, like Michel Petrone (Figure 1.6).

> So now I have a diagnosis, Hodgkin's disease. Let's call it cancer. I've heard of that.
> I know what it is—Fiona, a woman I live with is having chemotherapy for breast cancer. This is different, I'm told. They don't tell you that an 80% chance of cure means a 20% chance of death. You're left to work that one out for yourself. Death. Life is bad enough, that's what I thought. But who do I tell? Mum, I want to die. Hey, lover of mine, I think forever might be closer than I thought. Hi good friend, want to talk about euthanasia and writing a will?
> 'We're all in pain, why can't we share our pain?'
> Death and illness are almost taboo subjects even though we will all die eventually. Who isn't frightened and doesn't find it difficult to talk to someone they know might be dying? I wasn't prepared, neither were my family and friends. Who's going to help me, listen to me, understand me, be there for me—just for me. Not be frightened by my thoughts and feelings of having my life threatened, changed, and maybe dying at the end of it all anyway.

> Poem reproduced with permission of The Michele Angelo Petrone Foundation,
> <www.makingartpersonal.org>

The essential toolkit

Good clinical practice, in whatever profession or specialty field, integrates knowledge, skills, and attitudes. Unfortunately, we have seen many sad examples that have been taken before the General Medical Council, Nursing & Midwifery Council or other professional bodies where only one aspect of this triad has been practiced by the health care professional, to the cost of the patient. All three components are important for you to develop to provide good palliative care for your patients. For example:

1 **You will need to KNOW**

♦ about diseases and their natural history,

♦ about the potential causes of symptoms,

♦ about drugs and their safe use,

♦ about palliative care services and how to access them.

2 **You will need to be SKILLED in**

♦ communication,

♦ various technical procedures.

3 **In your ATTITUDE to patients, you should be**

♦ empathetic,

♦ holistic,

♦ compassionate.

In Chapter 8, we include the core competencies for palliative care as a tool for you to use to reflect on your current knowledge and level of confidence in your abilities, and to provide a clear understanding of what you need to develop. Perhaps you could fill in the questionnaire in Chapter 8 before reading any more of this book and then repeat it afterwards to see how much you've learned.

 SUMMARY BOX

Whichever branch of health care you choose to specialize in, you will be caring for people affected by advanced and terminal diseases. Patients with incurable illness can be professionally and personally challenging. Your professional competence in palliative care is not optional.

The core competences in end of life care (Chapter 8) will guide you in obtaining the appropriate knowledge, skills, and attitudes that will enable you to provide good care and gain a great deal of professional satisfaction.

KEY POINTS

In essence, patients and their carers may need:

- to be understood as the person they are, not the illness they have;
- their concerns listened to;
- information and discussion;
- support and counselling;
- symptom control;
- continuity of care and good team work;
- access to expert services;
- practical help.

Case history exercise: some thoughts on Mrs Jones

Of course, we can only guess what is on Mrs Jones's mind and what she might want from her doctor or other professionals. Only when we ask her will we really find out. Having some thoughts, however, may help you prepare for such a consultation, both in thinking about the answers and also in asking open questions that will help her tell you what she is thinking and feeling.

We usually use empathy (putting ourselves in her situation) to guess what might be on her mind, but we can also use the evidence base to guide us (i.e. what patients have told us in the past or told researchers) without, of course, making foolhardy assumptions about the individual patient.

Mrs Jones will probably want to know:

- what is happening to cause the swallowing problems;
- what it means about the progress of the MND;
- what can be done to improve things.

She will probably want her doctor to discuss with her:

- the treatment options;
- the detail of what they entail;
- the choices she can make.

She might want:

- to know how long her prognosis is;
- to know what she can expect to happen from now;
- to talk about telling her family;

- someone to help her with her feelings about her diagnosis and deterioration and the impact on her family and grandchildren;
- to be able to cry with someone who she does not have to look after;
- to reflect on the meaning of life and spiritual issues.

Her doctor and other health care professionals might want:

- to know what's important to her (to have/do/be and to not have/do/be) as she approaches the end of life;
- to learn more about her thoughts about decisions around the end of life, such as the use of antibiotics for pneumonia;
- to review the practical help that is needed and the arrangements for anticipating problems and preventing crises.

It is unlikely that the GP or most other professionals have much experience of MND and may wish to gain expert advice and support from the MND Association and the local palliative care service and specialist MND nurses.

References

1 **Neuberger, J.** (2013) *Independent Review of the Liverpool Care Pathway : More Care, Less Pathway*. London, Williams Lea.

2 *World Health Organization.* (2002) *National Cancer Control Programmes: Policies and Managerial Guidelines* (2nd edn). *Geneva: World Health Organization*

3 **Petrone, M.A.** (2003) *The Journey to Where? The Emotional Cancer Journey*. MAP Foundation.

4 **Munk, W.** (1887) *Euthanasia: Or Medical Treatment in Aid of an Easy Death*. London, Longmans, Green and Co.

5 **Nightingale, F.** (1860) *Notes on Nursing: What It Is and What It Is Not*. London, Harrison.

6 **Saunders, C.** (1967). The care of the terminal stages of cancer. *Annals of the Royal College of Surgeons of England*; **41** (Suppl.):162–9.

7 **Kubler-Ross, E.** (1969). *On Death and Dying*. Macmillan, New York.

8 **Parkes, C.M.** (1991). *Bereavement: Studies of Grief in Adult Life* (2nd edn). Penguin, London.

9 **Hinton, J.** (1972). *Dying* (2nd edn). Penguin, London.

10 **Department of Health.** (2008) *End of Life Care Strategy*. London, Department of Health.

11 **General Medical Council.** (2010) *Treatment and Care Towards the End of Life: Good Practice in Decision Making*. London, GMC.

12 **Bell, D.** (2010) GMC guidelines on end of life care. *BMJ*; **340**:c3231.

13 **Highet, G., Crawford, D., Murray, S.A., and Boyd, K.** (2014) Development and evaluation of the Supportive and Palliative Care Indicators Tool (SPICT): a mixed-methods study. *BMJ Supportive and Palliative Care*, online first article, doi:10.1136/bmjspcare–2013–000488.

14 **McCormack, P.** (1966) 'Crabbit old woman'. First published in Searle, C. (ed) (1973) *Elders*. London, Reality Press. (See also Bornat, J. (2005) *Empathy and Stereotype: The Work of a Popular Poem*. Available at <http://www.mchschurch.org/articles/Kate.pdf> accessed 29th May 2014.)

Further reading

Broyard, A. (1992) *Intoxicated By My Illness and Other Writings on Life and Death*. New York, Fawcett Columbine.

Faull, C., De Caestecker, S., Nicholson, A., and Black, F. (eds) (2012) *Handbook of Palliative Care* (3rd edn). New Jersey, Wiley-Blackwell.

Chapter 2

Palliative care assessment, communication, and challenging situations

Chapter 2

Palliative care assessment, communication, and challenging situations

The importance of communication

Holistic care, as discussed in the introduction on palliative care principles in Chapter 1, is fundamental to providing good palliative care. With this in mind, it is clear that an accurate assessment of a patient's needs, looking at the physical, emotional, social, and spiritual components, is essential. The WHO definition of palliative care[1] stresses the importance of 'impeccable assessment' (see section 'What is palliative care' in Chapter 1). Good communication is the basis for our success in assessing our patient. The quality of our communication also has a big impact on our patients' emotional health and physical symptoms, and poor communication is one of the main causes of patient complaints.[2,3] Patients and relatives are driven to complain when they do not feel they are listened to and when they do not feel that information has been shared with them honestly and in a sensitive and compassionate manner.

No-one sets out to be a poor communicator, and we all run the risk of underperforming at times. Also, when dealing with patients with life-threatening illnesses and their families, there are additional challenges we need to handle. To be a good communicator we need to develop awareness of the skills which help

 LEARNING EXERCISE

Think how you might feel and respond when faced with the following challenging situations:

- 'Is it serious?'
- 'How long have I got?'
- 'Don't tell him he's dying, he'll give up'.
- 'Why can't he be cured?'
- 'Can you end it for me?'

communication, the barriers to good communication, and strategies to help in challenging situations when dealing with people with life-threatening illnesses. This chapter aims to give you important practical communication tips to help you take a good history or holistic palliative care assessment which encourages patients and their families to discuss their concerns and help you deal with challenging conversations.

Palliative care assessment: the patient's story

Taking a palliative care history or making an assessment is, in its most basic form, a conversation between the health care professional and the patient. This is our chance to hear the patient's story and to gain a perspective on their physical, emotional, social, and spiritual needs. So it is important that the patient is offered the best opportunity to express their concerns and for these to be listened to. However, we know that patients often only tell us their physical concerns and other concerns, that are really important to them, remain undisclosed. Patients may assume we only want to hear about their physical problems unless *we* show that we want to know about all their various concerns.

As students, we are generally taught to assess by asking a series of specific questions in a structured format. Using conventions like this can be really helpful— we all know what is expected of us and where to find things in the notes. However, as you may have noticed, patients don't 'tell their story' according to our conventions and checklists, but give us information in a way that makes sense to them. One way of getting round this problem might be for you to take charge by interrupting and asking your questions anyway. Certainly, you would have a series of things to write in the notes, but would your behaviour have blocked communication between you and the patient? Would you have found out about the patient's concerns and, most importantly, would the patient feel listened to?

Alternatively, you could ask a good opening question and let the patient tell their story. As the consultation proceeds, with good, facilitative communication skills you will gain a picture of their concerns and can then seek clarification and attempt to explain things in a way that makes sense from the patient's

---

? THINK POINTS

Did you know that, on average, the health care professional interrupts the patient within 18 seconds of the consultation starting?

Did you know that, on average, 54% of patients' problems are not elicited during a consultation?

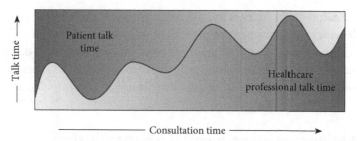

Figure 2.1 Rough representation of the time spent talking by a health care professional during a consultation using the structure we have suggested

perspective. This will mean that the patient does more of the talking initially. Then, you start to say more as the consultation goes on (see Figure 2.1). There is evidence that this approach works, you tend to get better-quality information, you understand patients more holistically, and, although we may worry that this will take longer, it actually takes less time.[4]

 LEARNING EXERCISE

Trying it out!

For the next patient you have to assess, let the patient tell their story and keep your writing to a minimum. Then write your assessment up in full afterwards. See what sort of information you get.

Eliciting the patient's concerns

Focusing on the patient's concerns rather than our agenda can feel a bit scary at first. We might worry; 'but what if I dry up or forget to ask a really important question and miss something?' Certainly, patients may not directly tell us what is wrong; instead, they may drop 'cues'. A cue is a hint, either verbal (e.g. repeated words or emotional phrases such as 'I'm worried') or non-verbal (e.g. tone of voice or expression), that something is wrong. Our job is to pick up on these cues. Patients are telling us they want to be listened to and, in order to identify their concerns, this is what we must do. It seems simple, but we not only need to listen but we also need to let patients *know* we are listening (active listening) in order to elicit their concerns and show that we care. Silverman et al.[5] identified communication behaviours which help facilitate patient disclosure of their concerns and also let them know that we are listening. By focusing on the patient's concerns, the interview should feel more like a 'purposeful discussion'

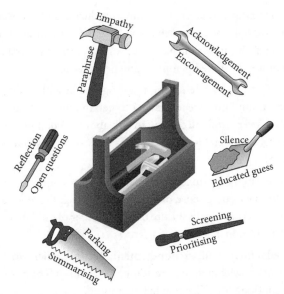

Figure 2.2 Communication tool-box of facilitation behaviours to help patients disclose their concerns

and less like an interrogation. The following are some facilitative behaviours which will help you to do this. Think of them as 'tools' to put in your 'tool box' (Figure 2.2).

- Use **open questions** to get patients talking and closed ones if you need to clarify something (see Table 2.1).

- Use **non-verbal communication** techniques to enhance disclosure and rapport (e.g. sitting not standing, good eye contact, nodding the head).

- **Reflection**; repeating back the patient's words.

- **Paraphrase**; similar to reflecting but using different words.

Table 2.1 Examples of open and closed questions

Examples of open questions	Examples of closed questions
'How are you today?'	'When did you have your endoscopy?'
'How can I help you?'	'Where exactly is your pain?'
'Tell me about your illness'.	'Would you say that you feel sick at meal times?'
'Tell me about you pain'.	'Are you worried about your wife?'
'You seem worried to me'.	'Do you take your tablet regularly?'
'Is there anything you want to ask me?'	'Can I talk about that at the next appointment?'

- Use **summarizing**; it is useful to summarize during and at the end of a consultation. This tells the patient that you have been listening, shows that you want to get it right, allows the patient to correct any misunderstanding, gives an opportunity for shared planning, and helps recall.

- **Empathy**; is a way of attempting to recognize how the patient is feeling and letting them know we are trying to get an appreciation of this, e.g. 'I can see this is very difficult for you to talk about'—*not* 'I understand', as we can never truly understand how another feels, even if we have had similar experiences.

- **Silence**; this often feels uncomfortable, but silences or pauses give a patient a chance to make some sense of what is happening. Evidence also suggests that these often precede disclosure of a concern or of difficult content, especially of an emotional nature.[3]

- **Acknowledgement and encouragement**; get the patient to expand on a subject by acknowledging (e.g. nodding, 'I see', 'mmm') or encouraging him or her to continue (e.g. 'Can you tell me more?').

- **Educated guess**; this is when the health care professional suggests what the patient is saying or feeling. If put tentatively, the patient can correct us if we are wrong and clarify the situation (e.g. 'Are you telling me you are frightened of going home?').

- **Parking**; this is when you put a concern to one side, to come back to it later, allowing you to continue to elicit concerns. Acknowledgement and empathy are important here to ensure that the patient doesn't feel ignored (e.g. 'That sounds difficult, I will come back to that. Before I do, can I just check if there are any other concerns?').

- **Screening questions**; these help you check you have elicited all the patient's concerns (e.g. 'Is there something else?').

- **Prioritizing**; this helps you find out which of the concerns is the most important to the patient (e.g. 'Which is the most important to you?').

- Be comfortable with **letting the patient take control**, even if this means them getting upset.

Use the 'learning exercise' to reflect on the effect of these skills in practice.

 LEARNING EXERCISE

Sit in on a patient interview with a colleague. Observe which of the facilitative skills are used, and note what sort of information they generate.

? **THINK POINT**

Getting the whole picture

Think of history taking or assessment as rather like a jigsaw. The pieces come to you at random, and the overall picture seems muddled at first, but as you go on, putting bits together, the true picture emerges.

Structuring the palliative care assessment

In order to have this 'purposeful discussion' about the patient's concerns and to 'put the pieces of the jigsaw together', it is useful to have a structure which helps and encourages patient involvement, ensures accurate understanding of the issues, and makes good use of time. There are many consultation models but one we have found useful in the palliative care setting is the Calgary-Cambridge consultation guide.[5] This model promotes an organized approach to patient assessment, consisting of five main sections that run in sequence throughout the discussion and incorporating structure and relationship building as a continuous thread throughout the consultation. The five sections are:

+ initiating the session,
+ gathering information,
+ physical examination,
+ explanation and planning,
+ closing the session (see Figure 2.3).

Further information, particularly regarding application in practice, can be found at <www.gp-training.net/training/communication_skills/calgary/index.htm>

It important to note that 'explanation and planning' occurs in this model when all of the 'information gathering' has been done. As health care professionals, we want to help our patients and often try and give information and problem solve before we have identified all the patient's concerns. We do this with the best of intentions, as we want to help and 'make it right' as soon as we can. However, by trying to 'fix' things too soon, we might block the patient from telling us something important. Also, there are some things we cannot 'fix' for the patient or family. Some of the skills in your 'tool-box'—screening, parking, and prioritizing—are particularly useful to help elicit all of the patient's concerns and prevent giving information and problem solving too soon. Figure 2.4 shows how these can be used to help us see the full jigsaw puzzle.

When we do need to give information and plan, we need to do so in a way that is clear and unambiguous for it to be remembered and understood. Remember,

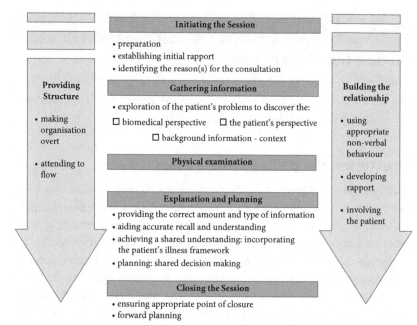

Figure 2.3 Calgary-Cambridge Model (Silverman et al. 2013[5])

Reproduced with permission from Silverman, J.D. et al., *Skills for Communicating with Patients*, Third Edition, Radcliffe Medical Press, Oxford, UK, Copyright © 2013.

patients hear and take in information more effectively if it is given in small amounts and we check out their understanding before moving on. The 'Learning Exercise' may help you develop this skill in your practice.

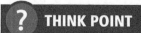 **THINK POINT**

Information giving

Think of information giving as 'chunking and checking'. This involves delivering information in small amounts, then stopping and checking that the patient has taken it in and understood.

 LEARNING EXERCISE

Trying it out!

Next time you have to give information to a patient, try slowing the pace down by 'chunking and checking'. Then, consider what effect this may have had on the patient's understanding.

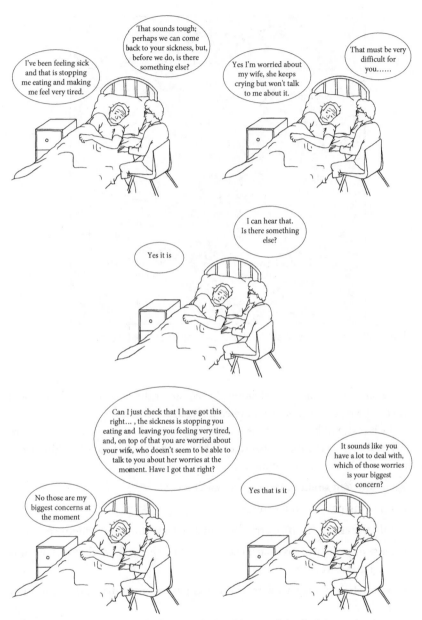

Figure 2.4 Using screening, parking, and prioritizing to elicit all of the patient's concerns

Blocking behaviours and barriers

Blocking behaviours stop patients telling you about their concerns and may be used by us either intentionally or unintentionally. We may adopt these behaviours as a result of anxieties about caring for someone at the end of life or the challenges

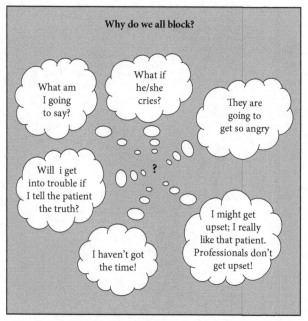

Figure 2.5 Reasons why health care professionals use blocking behaviours

of the care environment (see Figure 2.5). Whatever the reason, these behaviours will form barriers to good communication with patients.

Much research has been done in this area, but perhaps the work by Maguire and Faulkner[6] is the most celebrated. They categorized various blocking techniques used by doctors and nurses:

* Getting into **small talk** and personal 'chit chat'.

* **Ignoring** patients' questions.

* **Jollying along**: 'Don't worry about that, at least you're going home today'.

* **False or premature reassurance**: saying it will be 'alright' when it is obvious to all that it won't.

* **Normalizing**: suggesting that something is common may indicate it is not important.

* **Switching the topic**: patient: 'Am I dying?'; nurse: 'How is your breathing today?'.

* **Switching the focus**: patient: 'I'm struggling to manage at home'; nurse: 'How is your wife coping?'.

* **Passing the buck**: 'I don't know, you had better ask the consultant'.

◆ Use of **jargon**: patient: 'Is it cancer?'; doctor: 'You've got an adenocarcinoma of the right main bronchus'.

The shocking truth is that all of us will use these techniques occasionally, without knowing it. We need to become more aware of them and be mindful of the sort of situations when we might use them. In this way, we can limit the impact on our patients.

 THINK POINT

Styles of communicators

In her observational work of nurses caring for patients with cancer on an oncology ward, Wilkinson[7] identified four styles of communicators:

◆ *Facilitators* consistently use facilitative skills like the ones described in the tool-box, to ensure their communication is patient-centred and to allow patients to disclose their concerns.

◆ *Ignorers* consistently miss or block patient cues by the use of blocking behaviours.

◆ *Informers* give information or opinions when not appropriate.

◆ *Mixers* do a mixture of facilitation and blocking behaviours.

Use the following 'Learning Exercise' to develop your skills in reflecting on interactions with patients. This will help you embed communication skills that are most effective for patients.

 LEARNING EXERCISE

Observe a colleague undertaking a patient interview. Are they predominantly using skills which 'facilitate', 'inform', 'ignore', or are a mixture?

Handling challenging situations

General principles

Much of what we've talked about so far applies equally in more difficult situations, only the emotion, and therefore the stakes, tend to be higher in the circumstances listed below:

◆ breaking bad news

◆ giving a poor prognosis

- discussing dying
- being asked to hide the truth (collusion)
- the angry patient/family
- the request for help to die

These difficult conversations are often related to discussing death and dying with patients and their families, and are usually associated with dealing with strong emotions. Our approach to these conversations will be unique to us and the particular situation. In general, however, such consultations work best when they follow a similar pattern to the one outlined in Figure 2.6. Not that communication is ever this structured—thank goodness! However, this gives us a framework on which to base our conversations.

We can't, of course, be there to tell you what words to use, or consider the infinite number of possible variations on these themes. You need to develop your own style with which you feel comfortable. All we can say is that you will be in these positions, that how you handle them makes a difference, and that it is never easy.

There are other situations that are also challenging, but these difficult conversations are the ones that tend to give us most anxiety and are associated with feelings of discomfort and inadequacy. Much of our success in these sorts of consultations depends on our sensitivity and confidence. A textbook like this cannot teach these skills, all we can do is to give you some guidance. That is not to say that these skills cannot be learned—they can. Readers may have an opportunity to undertake communication skills training, either through role play or video work. We urge you to take these opportunities, even if you really feel uncomfortable about it. It is your chance to practise!

 THINK POINT

Quotes from professionals about breaking bad news

'It's probably the most important clinical thing I do. It's got to set the framework for the treatment'.

'If the patient has been alive for 50 years, they don't need to be told that they're dying in a minute'.

'The doctor usually gives the bad news initially, but when I go back to the patient, to see how they are, I feel like it is me giving the bad news when I confirm what they have been told. That's why it is so important we work together as a team'.

 LEARNING EXERCISE

When you are next talking to a patient who has been given bad news, ask how it was done and what it felt like to receive the news.

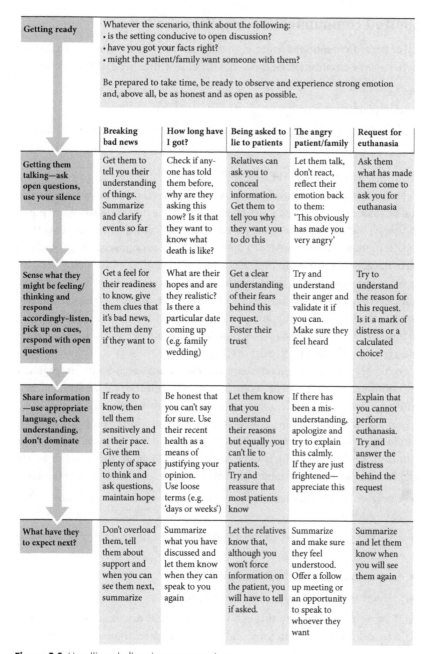

Getting ready	Whatever the scenario, think about the following: • is the setting conducive to open discussion? • have you got your facts right? • might the patient/family want someone with them? Be prepared to take time, be ready to observe and experience strong emotion and, above all, be as honest and as open as possible.				
	Breaking bad news	**How long have I got?**	**Being asked to lie to patients**	**The angry patient/family**	**Request for euthanasia**
Getting them talking—ask open questions, use your silence	Get them to tell you their understanding of things. Summarize and clarify events so far	Check if anyone has told them before, why are they asking this now? Is it that they want to know what death is like?	Relatives can ask you to conceal information. Get them to tell you why they want you to do this	Let them talk, don't react, reflect their emotion back to them: 'This obviously has made you very angry'	Ask them what has made them come to ask you for euthanasia
Sense what they might be feeling/thinking and respond accordingly–listen, pick up on cues, respond with open questions	Get a feel for their readiness to know, give them clues that it's bad news, let them deny if they want to	What are their hopes and are they realistic? Is there a particular date coming up (e.g. family wedding)	Get a clear understanding of their fears behind this request. Foster their trust	Try and understand their anger and validate it if you can. Make sure they feel heard	Try to understand the reason for this request. Is it a mark of distress or a calculated choice?
Share information —use appropriate language, check understanding, don't dominate	If ready to know, then tell them sensitively and at their pace. Give them plenty of space to think and ask questions, maintain hope	Be honest that you can't say for sure. Use their recent health as a means of justifying your opinion. Use loose terms (e.g. 'days or weeks')	Let them know that you understand their reasons but equally you can't lie to patients. Try and reassure that most patients know	If there has been a mis-understanding, apologize and try to explain this calmly. If they are just frightened—appreciate this	Explain that you cannot perform euthanasia. Try and answer the distress behind the request
What have they to expect next?	Don't overload them, tell them about support and when you can see them next, summarize	Summarize what you have discussed and let them know when they can speak to you again	Let the relatives know that, although you won't force information on the patient, you will have to tell if asked.	Summarize and make sure they feel understood. Offer a follow up meeting or an opportunity to speak to whoever they want	Summarize and let them know when you will see them again

Figure 2.6 Handling challenging conversations

Limited communication: another challenge

All of the aforementioned assumes that the patient can enter into open discussion. In some circumstances, this is not the case, either because the patient:

♦ is too ill;

♦ is unconscious or dying;

♦ doesn't share a common language/culture with the health care professional;

♦ is confused;

♦ or does not wish to discuss the issues you want to cover.

In all such situations, communication will, of course, be compromised. But it is still beholden on us to make every effort to overcome these problems, accepting, of course, that we should respect a patient's wish to avoid talking about certain topics. In many cases, a barrier to open communication means using others to fill in the gaps (e.g. carers, interpreters, other professionals). In so doing, we have to make judgements as to the strength and validity of advocacy of each of these sources. This often means asking more than one person for their input. This will confirm the impression we come to, so that we and the team can continue to act in the patient's best interest (see section 'A good death needs decisions: what are the 'right'' decisions for patients? in Chapter 4).

For those patients who do not share a common language with us, the problem of communication may be complicated by cultural misunderstandings. Although familiarity with different cultural health beliefs might give us an advantage in understanding patients of a different ethnic group, we must be careful not to make assumptions about a patient's beliefs because of his or her ethnic group. The key thing is to be confident in the belief that it is fine to ask and to acknowledge uncertainty. The following are some core skills in this area:

♦ Check on the pronunciation of your patient's name and how he or she wishes to be addressed.

♦ Discover patients' ideas, concerns, and expectations. That means listening to what they say.

♦ Be non-judgemental about ideas and beliefs.

♦ Demonstrate interest, concern, and respect.

♦ Behave with sensitivity throughout the physical examination. Make sure you seek permission to look and touch and check how the patient feels about it.

♦ Incorporate their health understanding in your explanations.

♦ Have a negotiating approach to management.

SUMMARY BOX

Communication underpins our success in assessing patients in palliative care. Using your skills effectively will enable you to identify the patients' concerns. Some might argue that it is wrong or unrealistic to expect health care professionals always to have discussions or to consult with patients and their carers in the way outlined in this chapter, either because it seems unnecessary, as the issues are straightforward, or because workload and environmental issues make it difficult . However, it is important to reflect on your own skills and not underestimate when you might block patients and families from telling you their concerns, especially in challenging situations. There are useful ways of handling these challenging situations (e.g. breaking bad news). Remember, good communication is not an optional extra. You can learn to communicate well.

 KEY POINTS

Undertaking a palliative care assessment from the patients' perspective will require you to:

- have a 'tool-box' of communication skills at your fingertips that you can call upon as needed;
- know when to use different skills in different situations;
- be able to recognize when your approach is not working, and know how to change to a more effective style.

References

1. **World Health Organization.** (2002) *National Cancer Control Programmes: Policies and Managerial Guidelines* (2nd edn). Geneva, World Health Organization.
2. **Healthcare Commission.** (2008) *Spotlight on Complaints*. London, Commission for Healthcare Audit and Inspection.
3. **Parliamentary & Health Service Ombudsman.** (2011) *Listening and Learning: The Ombudsman Review of Complaint Handling by the NHS in England 2010–11*. London, The Stationery Office.
4. **Levinson, W., Gorawara-Bhat, R., and Lamb, J.** (2000) A study of patient clues and physician responses in primary care and surgical settings. *JAMA*; **284**:1429–33.
5. **Silverman, J.D., Kutz, S.M., and Draper, J.** (2013) *Skills for Communicating with Patients* (3rd edn). Oxford, Radcliffe Medical Press.

6. **Maguire, P. and Faulkner, A.** (1994) *Talking to Cancer Patients and Their Relatives.* Oxford, Oxford University Press.

7. **Wilkinson, S.M.** (1991) Factors which influence how nurses communicate with cancer patients. *J Adv Nurs*; **16**:677–88.

Further reading

Buckman, R. (2005) Breaking bad news: the S-P-I-K-E-S strategy. *Community Oncology*; 2:138–42.

De Caestecker, S. (2012) Communication skills in palliative care. **In** Faull, C., de Caestecker, S., Nicholson, A., and Black, F. (eds) *Handbook of Palliative Care* (3rd edn). New Jersey, Wiley-Blackwell.

Dunphy J. *Communication in palliative care*, London Radcliffe, 2011.

Fallowfield, L. (2011). Communication with the patient and family in palliative medicine. **In** Hanks G, Cherny N, Christakis N, Fallon M, Kassa D, Portenoy K. *Oxford Textbook of Palliative Medicine* (4th edn). Oxford, Oxford university Press.

Kai, J. (ed) (2005) *PROCEED: Professionals Responding to Ethnic Diversity and Cancer.* London, Cancer Research UK.

Kurtz, S., Silverman, J., and Draper, J. (2005) *Teaching and Learning Communication Skills in Medicine* (2nd edn). Oxford, Radcliffe Publishing.

Pettifer, A. (2013) Responding to questions about the end of life. **In** De Souza, J. and Pettifer, A. *End-of-life Nursing Care: A Guide for Best Practice*. London, Sage Publications.

Psychosocial and spiritual components of care

Psychosocial and spiritual components of care

Psychosocial and spiritual components of care and why they matter

Health care is about both understanding illness and understanding people. Each aspect is vitally important if we want to be good health care practitioners. However, our training often concentrates on the necessity of mastering the complexity of disease and the array of technical skills we can utilize; in addition, there is a pressure to complete physical care tasks in practice. This emphasis makes it harder to always see the value in considering the wider context of the disease experience for our patients.

An impending death, like almost no other situation in health care, reminds us of the importance of understanding people at the same time as we manage their disease. Whilst we can never truly understand, we can try and imagine what it would like to 'be in another person's shoes' (see empathy in section 'Eliciting the patients concerns' in Chapter 2).

Did you know that if you can appreciate the patient's perspective when he or she is ill, you are:

+ more likely to be effective at making accurate assessments of patients;
+ more likely to succeed in controlling patients' physical symptoms;
+ more likely to feel that the patient values your help—one of the most positive rewards in health care;
+ more likely to diagnose and treat depression;
+ less likely to make mistakes and have complaints made about you;
+ less likely to feel burned out.

Use the following 'learning exercises' to help you reflect upon the impact of a life- threatening diagnosis and what patients want from their health care professionals at this difficult time.

LEARNING EXERCISE

The challenge—it's about you

You can do this on your own or with a fellow student or colleague.

1. Write down all the things that are important in your life (e.g. family, friends, your hopes for the future).

2. Now imagine you were told that you had a diagnosis, the average prognosis of which was 12 months.

3. Cross off the list the things you will not be able to do and imagine (or tell your friend) what that feels like. How would you want health professionals to help you?

 LEARNING EXERCISE

What do patients want from you?

When you next see a patient and you have the time, try asking the following (it can be any patient):

+ Think of a health care professional you have found to be most helpful. What was it that made them good at their job?

+ Think of a health care professional you have found to be least helpful (no names). What was it that made them least helpful?

+ What do you think a health care professional should be like when looking after someone who is dying?

For some, this chapter will be inherently interesting; we hope you enjoy it. To the more sceptical, we challenge you to read it, and yourself answer this question: 'What sort of doctor/nurse/ allied health professional will your dying patients need?'

Dame Cicely Saunders (see section 'A little bit of history' in Chapter 1) asked a patient this same question:

> I once asked a dying patient what he wanted to see most in the people who were caring for him. He replied: 'For someone to look as if they are trying to understand me'. We may often fail, but they will be comforted and helped by any sincere effort and nothing else will take its place.[1]

> ## Box 3.1 PEPSI COLA aide memoire for assessment of a patient's needs
>
> | | |
> |---|---|
> | P—Physical | C—Control |
> | E—Emotional | O—Out of hours |
> | P—Personal | L—Living with your illness |
> | S—Social support | A—After-care |
> | I—Information and communication | |
>
> Reproduced with permission from National Gold Standards Framework Centre, *The PEPSI COLA Aide-memoire*, Copyright © 2014 National Gold Standards Framework Centre.

So how can I improve?

Developing our attitude in this area is a lifelong task for us all. There is much talk about the need for us to show care and compassion as a result of complaints about NHS care.[2,3] We need to be able to constantly reflect and learn from our experience and strive to be better in our role as a consequence (easier said than done). How we each do this depends on many influences, and one chapter in one book can only hope to have a very modest effect. However, we hope that we can give you an introduction to some of the methods and ways of thinking that could help you to be more effective in trying to understand our patients.

Why is holistic care so important?

The term 'holisitic' originates from the Greek word 'holos' meaning 'all, whole, entire, total'. As such, this implies we need to understand our patients as a whole person, including spiritual, social, emotional, and physical factors, to appreciate the impact of their illness on them. Each of these areas should be considered when assessing and caring for our patients. Holistic care is central to the philosophy of palliative care. Several useful tools are available to support us in holistic assessment. One example is the PEPSI COLA aide memoire (see Box 3.1), designed as part of the Gold Standards Framework for palliative care.[4] The accompanying guidance document presents useful cue questions and suggests relevant resources to assist practitioners. You can access the Pepsi Cola Aide Memoire and guidance document at <www.goldstandardsframework.org.uk>

Ways people react to knowing they are dying soon

The 'case history exercise' that follows is but one patient's story illustrating the extent of the psychosocial and spiritual needs of patients who are dying. Of course, each patient you look after will have his or her own story and resulting needs. We must strive to try and appreciate how they and their families are feeling. On the face of it, this seems complex. However, some emotions can be reasonably predicted and should be considered when interviewing patients; namely, fear, sadness, and anger. The drivers for these emotions and the extent they are experienced vary from person to person and reflect their unique circumstances and personality.

 CASE HISTORY EXERCISE

Colin was 54 when he died, 3 years after his diagnosis of renal cell carcinoma was made. He was a self-employed management consultant who had separated from Karen because of several infidelities. She, however, was his main carer in his last months. He had three children—Judith, studying sports science; Claire, a nanny; and Joseph, who was doing his A levels. His mother lived alone and suffered from Alzheimer's disease. Think about each of these characters and try to imagine the issues:

♦ Colin's views of his own, premature death; his feeling about his relationship with Karen; and his thoughts about his mother.

♦ Karen's feelings about her relationship with Colin; her thoughts about her future role and responsibilities.

♦ The children's feelings about their father's death and his past infidelities.

It's little wonder many patients and their carers will be frightened and suffer as a consequence.

Figure 3.1 illustrates some of the aspects of life considered important by most of us; the very things that 'make us tick'. It is how each patient views and copes with each of these components, when facing the end of their life, that drives their emotions and subsequent behaviour. At the same time as the patient is tussling with such thoughts, his or her relatives and friends are likely to be concerned about similar issues.

Understanding what is important to patients and their families in the past, now, and in the future will give us a clearer idea of why they feel and behave as they do. Only then do we stand a chance of *really* helping them with their worries and concerns.

Spirituality

Spirituality may include someone's religious beliefs but it is not necessarily, and certainly not solely, about religion. Sometimes, we are not really sure what it is

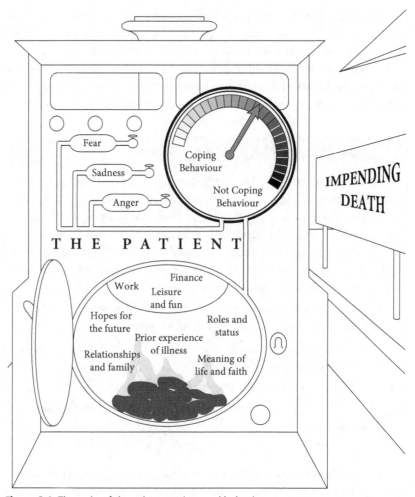

Figure 3.1 The train of thought, emotion, and behaviour

and how it relates to health care, and indeed there is a clear indication that we are not very good at broaching the subject and assessing what spiritual needs patients may have.[5] So, how do we define it and how can we provide spiritual support?

 LEARNING EXERCISE

Consider which, if any, of the definitions in Figure 3.2 correspond to your own thoughts on spirituality. Then write your own definition.

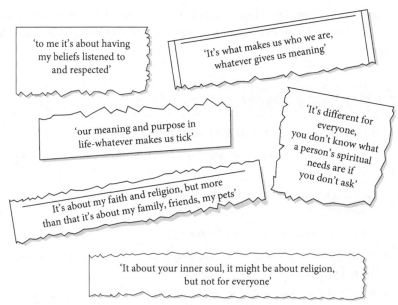

Figure 3.2 Some thoughts of health care professionals on spirituality and spiritual support

Much of the time, we may take these things for granted, but how does illness change this? This may, of course, depend on the illness. If we have a simple illness (e.g. a common cold) our spiritual needs may not be so important to us. However, the prospect of death is likely to mean that spiritual needs play a much bigger part and are more important for our patients. If we are not asking patients and their families about them, we may be missing an important aspect of how we need to care for them.

We are all familiar with the emotions of sadness, fear, and anger, but few of us have felt these emotions in the same way as someone facing their own death. Patients differ in how they cope. Some take their impending death seemingly in their stride; others fluctuate in their ability to cope; and some struggle to retain any control. The forces that influence how patients cope are diverse to say the least. When speaking to patients, we must give them an opportunity to express their feelings at a pace they are happy with. Learning to listen and showing we care enough to try and understand is a central skill of being effective in our role. Not only will people feel so much better for feeling we are caring and compassionate, you will probably find your work more rewarding. In the sections 'The importance of communication' and 'Handling challenging situations' in Chapter 2, we outlined some of the skills needed to explore these issues with patients in a way that is effective.

The following 'Learning Exercise' may help you think further about aspects of psychosocial and spiritual care and the possible challenges for health professionals.

 LEARNING EXERCISE

What is it like to look after the dying?

Choose a colleague you respect and ask him or her the following sorts of questions:

- Can you remember the last dying patient you looked after, where things went well?
- What sort of person was the patient?
- When you were looking after the patient, how well did you understand what they wanted?
- What did it feel like to look after this patient?

After you've heard the answers, consider the depth at which your colleague knew the patient's psychosocial and spiritual background.

The theory and how it helps

One way of helping us to be effective in our understanding of the psychosocial and spiritual needs of our patients, is to be familiar with some of the theory that can explain what is going on (see Box 3.2). If we are able to stand outside of the process and analyse it, then we can:

- make better sense of the emotions and behaviour we observe;
- feel that the consultation is not out of control and that the patient's emotions and behaviour do not overwhelm us;
- better predict what is going on and so be more effective in how we offer help.

Different disciplines have contributed to our understanding of how patients' feelings and behaviour can be understood (Figure 3.3). There is a lot written on this subject and it is beyond the scope of this book to give you a very detailed account of all relevant theories. What we hope is that by showing you a sample of some of the most quoted work, you will be able to appreciate the effectiveness of this approach in everyday practice. After you have read about the theories, use the 'Learning Exercise' to help apply these to your practice.

Box 3.2 Theories and holidays—an analogy to understanding

Imagine planning an exciting holiday to a place you're never visited. How would you find out about where you were going? You'd go to different sources to get the information; road map, globe, travel guide, the web, a well-travelled friend, etc. Each source would tell you something true about the place, albeit from slightly different perspectives. The same could be said for theories that explain patient's emotions and behaviour. Each theory gives us a clearer understanding of what is going on. No one theory gives us all the answers, and some are more useful than others in different circumstances. However, they can all help guide us as we try to make sense of our patients.

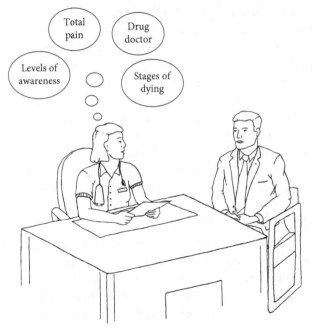

Figure 3.3 Using key theories and models in the real world of interaction with patients

Total pain

Dame Cecily Saunders (the founder of the modern hospice movement in the United Kingdom; see section 'A little bit of hisory' in Chapter 1) devised the concept of total pain[6.] Classically, pain is understood physiologically in terms of

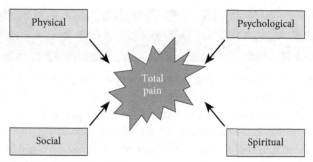

Figure 3.4 The theory of total pain

a noxious stimulus causing an unpleasant sensation; and this is true. However, the experience of pain is more complex than just a physical sensation and it is important to view it holistically (Figure 3.4). A patient's pain will be worse if they also have powerful negative emotions, such as anxiety, anger, and depression. In fact, for those that struggle to express their distress, using the language of pain can be helpful. This concept of total pain can be especially useful when assessing patients whose pain presents atypically, or where the response to analgesics is inconsistent or incomplete. It is important not to dismiss this pain as unreal or 'in the mind'; it isn't, and must be taken seriously, requiring active management. Only, this management might not mean the escalation of analgesic drugs, but allowing the patient's distress to be recognized and understood, and, if appropriate, managed by non-pharmacological methods. The total pain concept can help us to assess pain and other symptoms by considering their relationship to a range of emotional, spiritual, and practical issues.

Stages or tasks of dying

In her often-quoted work, following her observations of dying patients, Kubler-Ross[7] describes five stages of dying These stages may be experienced sequentially, with individuals moving from stage to stage. However, often patients tend to jump around the stages, back and forth. Some patients seem to reach 'acceptance' very quickly, whereas others struggle to reach this point and never get there. The five stages are:

1. **Denial**: avoiding the harsh reality when given a terminal diagnosis.
2. **Anger**: the 'Why me?' response. The anger can be directed at family or friends, or at us as health care professionals.
3. **Bargaining**: the patient attempts to ward off the inevitable by making a deal with the professional, family, or God. 'Surely doctor, if I have this big operation I'm bound to be cured?'

4. **Depression**: the realization of the forthcoming loss of life results in feelings of depression, guilt, anxiety, and hopelessness.

5. **Acceptance**: the end of the struggle. The patient has generally transcended the previous four stages of emotional adaptation.

Unfortunately, the title 'stages' suggests a mechanistic approach and has been criticized for being too restrictive. An alternative 'task-based approach' has been proposed by Corr,[8] in which he suggests that the dying patient needs to complete the following 'tasks' in order to cope:

1. Satisfying physical needs and minimizing distress.

2. Maximizing psychological security, autonomy, and richness in living.

3. Sustaining and enhancing significant relationships.

4. Identifying, developing, or reaffirming sources of spiritual strength and fostering hope.

Corr[8] argues that for health professionals who are dealing with dying, it is helpful to think of these tasks in order to consider whether and what assistance is required in completing them.

Contexts of death awareness

Glaser and Strauss[9] and, later, Timmermans[10] have described how patients, professionals, and family may and may not share diagnostic and prognostic information according to the 'contexts of awareness' groups described in Figure 3.5.

Obviously, the ideal position for the health care professionals and most patients is active, open awareness, enabling acknowledgement and frank discussion of the facts of dying. Although all contexts are emotionally exacting, open awareness gives the greatest likelihood of the death the patient most wishes, as it is possible to have honest discussions about those wishes.

Drug doctor

Putting aside this unfortunate ambiguous phrase Balint[11] has been hugely influential. His work in the late 1950s resulted in the concept of a 'drug doctor'. He felt that one of the most frequently used and powerful agents within the consultation was the doctor (and, most probably, other professionals). Patients can gain great benefit, or indeed great harm, from how the health care professional interacts with them. This can be a useful concept to hold onto when speaking with patients, especially in those discussions when we do not seem to be doing anything but listen. You will be surprised how much being listened to really helps. Your interaction with a patient can have a very big therapeutic effect and you can maximize this through your excellent communication skills and holistic approach.

Closed awareness	Suspended awareness	Mutual pretence	Open awareness
The patient does not recognize they are dying, but everyone else does.	The patient suspects what others know and attempts to verify this, but staff and family avoid the questioning.	All the players in the game (patient, family and staff) are aware of the impending death, but all continue as if they are not.	Everyone is aware of the impending death and this may be acknowledged in interactions.

Suspended open awareness	Uncertain awareness	Active open awareness
The truth is given but then blocked out by patients and their kin.	Patients and professionals selectively retain good information. Ignoring more pessimistic news. Medical uncertainty is used to draw a veil over the negatives.	The patient and family understand the prognosis and actively try to come to terms with it. The patient no longer hopes for recovery.

Figure 3.5 Awareness of dying theory

Source: data from Timmermans, S., Dying awareness: the theory of awareness revisited, *Social Health and Illness*, Volume 16, Number 3, pp. 322–337, Copyright © Basil Blackwell Ltd/Editorial Board 1994.

 LEARNING EXERCISE

Theory and practice

Next time you're observing a colleague assessing a patient, especially in a challenging situation, see if any of the theories apply. When you are more skilled, you may be able to think of some of these theories when listening to patients yourself. At the end, ask yourself 'Does it help to think like this?'.

Focusing on feelings

If we are to really try and appreciate what patients think and feel, we need to be skilled at getting them to share their psychosocial and spiritual concerns with us. We have to be comfortable about taking a patient-centred history or assessment,

> ## Box 3.3 Quotes from patients
>
> 'They were all very nice, very wonderful, but I realized afterwards that nobody told me anything'. (Female heart failure patient)
>
> 'He never told her the cancer was in her arm as well, but he told me and he said "I'll leave it with you to tell her"'. (Husband of breast cancer patient)
>
> 'But no-one asked me how I was feeling. They don't get it. I'm going to die'. (Male interstitial lung disease patient)

talking about what worries them, and listening, and be able to observe emotional distress. Only then will we be able to make accurate assessments of patients' needs and give the high-quality care to which we all aspire. What is more, inaccurate assessments not only cause patients to suffer but they also waste time and resources and lead to complaints.[3] The section 'The importance of communication skills' in Chapter 2 has discussed this and some of the specific communications skills required in palliative care . Our ability to demonstrate empathy will be key. However, communicating effectively with patients requires more than the knowledge of what you ought to say and do. It also requires you to have skills that need to be practised. Just to give you an idea of how important it is to get this right, have a look at what patients say (see Box 3.3).

Whatever stage we are in our careers, we gain in experience as we see more and more patients. But this does not mean we necessarily get better at communicating. What we need to do is to be able to reflect on how we communicate in a way that promotes positive change. The easiest way of doing this is to take advantage of the increasing number of communication skills courses available. Research[12-14] suggests the most effective methods usually involve the rather scary business of being observed by your peers (either on video or in role play) and getting feedback from a skilled tutor. Most of us, especially as beginners in this sort of situation, find it intimidating. But it really will make a difference (see Box 3.4).

Barriers to good psychosocial and spiritual care and what stops us caring

None of us wants to be unkind when dealing with patients, but most of us probably will be. Not all the time or at a level that causes significant distress, but it happens more than we might think. This is not because we want to be horrible, but because we are human. Only when we recognize this truth do we stand any chance of protecting our patients and ourselves from underperformance. By

---

Box 3.4 Quotes about being taught communications skills

'My surgeon had been on one of those courses and he said he tried to encourage others to do so, but it seems that those who really need it don't *think* they need it'. (Female breast cancer patient)

'I was not keen to do this at first, but found it really beneficial in the end'. (Medical student)

'Role plays are sometimes embarrassing, but always good'. (GP)

'I was so scared I wouldn't know what to say but everyone was so supportive and I have learnt so much'. (Nurse)

'As a physio I never really had any communication skills training. I wish I had done this course sooner'. (Physiotherapist)

---

appreciating the pressures we are under and how we behave with patients, we can then develop ways of minimizing the damage.

External barriers

Our work environment has a significant impact on how we function. We have to deal with a range of pressures that can result in us not helping the dying as much as we would like or they would need. By recognizing these pressures, we can go some way to anticipating when we might be underperforming:

- **Workload and prioritization**: it is little wonder that if we are required to work in a way that demands us to process patients at speed, then we run the risk of ignoring everything but the immediate and necessary. And rarely are the psychosocial and spiritual needs considered immediate and necessary by professionals. Most of us, to a greater or lesser extent, fall foul of this most days. The danger is not recognizing that we are doing this and consequently developing a way of working that routinely excludes patients' psychosocial concerns.

- **Colleagues**: even if you have a well-developed appreciation of the importance of psychosocial and spiritual needs, if you work with colleagues who don't share these views, then your efforts in this area can, at best, go unrewarded and, at worst, be openly criticized. It is difficult, but crucial, to be strong and maintain you own force of conviction in what you know is good care.

- **Teamwork**: good psychosocial and spiritual care depends on team members collaborating in an atmosphere that promotes understanding of patients. If you work in a more isolated way, then opportunities to help patients will be missed.

- **Place**: for patients to tell us their worries, they need to feel confident and comfortable. Many of the places we are required to work are not conducive to such an atmosphere (e.g. a busy ward with little privacy).

Internal barriers

There are other barriers, closer to home, that might also stop us performing at our best. These include:

- **Tiredness**: if we are physically or emotionally exhausted, then we may have little left to give to our patients. There is a paradox here: the more we give to our patients, the higher the potential risk to our own emotional well-being. What we obviously need to know is where the balance lies for us and when we are getting exhausted.

- **Work ethic**: throughout our training, we are rewarded for hard work. Taking a break or saying 'no' is considered, by some, as a sign of weakness and failure. All you have to ask yourself is, 'Who are you failing if you get exhausted?'.

- **Professional attitudes**: some of our training leads us to believe that the psychosocial and spiritual aspects of patient care are not our job. We're in this business to cure disease after all—aren't we? (We know *you* don't think like this!)

- **Confidence**: if you feel underconfident in how to help people with psychosocial and spiritual problems, you may handle this by trying to ignore the issues. And given the power we have during our conversations with patients, we are well able to avoid areas that make us feel uncomfortable. Hopefully, with experience and practice, you should overcome this problem.

- **Personal experience**: we are people too! We will, at some times in our lives, undergo life events that stretch our coping strategies. This will affect our work to a greater or lesser degree. Sometimes, for instance after a loss and period of grief, we are in a better position to understand our patient's predicament. Conversely, our emotional reserves can be stretched to the point where it is hard to accommodate the distress of others.

- **Illness**: our own physical or mental illness can also impact on how we behave towards our patients and colleagues. Do not underestimate this.

Box 3.5 Risk factors for burn out

Does any of this sound like you?

+ Perfectionist
+ Overly conscientious
+ Like pleasing people
+ Need to control others
+ Great sense of responsibility
+ Chronic self-doubt
+ Uncomfortable with praise

If so, look out—BURN OUT ALERT!

How to look after yourself—avoiding burn out

'But it won't happen to me' we hear you say. You're probably right. But the truth is that we are all at risk and some of us are more at risk than others (Box 3.5). Failing to be aware of the rigours of our job and life make us especially vulnerable to burn out. So how do we protect ourselves? The following will help:

+ Recognize when you are stressed and what makes you feel like this.
+ Talk to colleagues. We all have a quick moan or share stories about difficult work situations. Doing this with someone who will listen, helps. You might be surprised how much of this goes on (see the following 'Learning exercise').
+ Don't lose your sense of humour.
+ Take breaks and learn how you best relax. Do something other than work.
+ Learn to say 'no'. Obviously, we have a job of work to do and we aspire to do it to a high standard. Also, as professionals who are reasonably rewarded for what we do, we have at times to go the extra mile for our patients. However, this should not mean saying 'yes' to extra tasks that are not necessarily advantageous to our patients, or to us. You should not feel guilty about this.
+ Plan whenever possible.
+ Remember, how you work is under your own control. Health care has the advantages of a variety of work patterns; we have to be brave enough to choose the one we really want for ourselves.
+ Identify your support network. Who are the people from whom you get support in different circumstances (see Figure 3.6)?

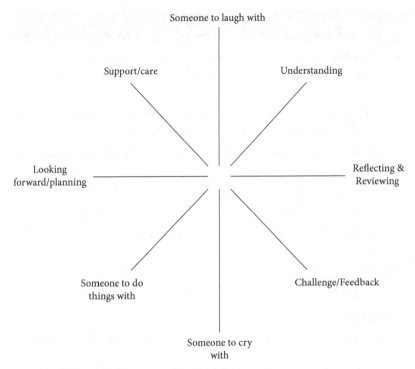

Figure 3.6 Framework for a support network [15]
Image: Copyright © Hilary Cotton, developed from work by Tom Boydell, Rosemary Warner, Rob West and Hilary Cotton. Reprinted with permission of the author.

 LEARNING EXERCISE

Next time you're sitting in the staff room, have a listen to what people are talking about.

♦ Are they listening to each other's worries?

♦ Are they being supportive?

SUMMARY BOX

Holistic care is fundamental to palliative care. You will need to consider the psychosocial and spiritual elements when caring for your patients, as well as the physical aspects. You also need to recognize when and what might prevent you from exploring these areas with patients and families. In this way, you can care for the 'whole person'.

KEY POINTS

- To be a health care professional, and especially to do that well, we need to be able to try and understand people as well as we understand their illness.

- Listening to and caring for people's psychosocial and spiritual needs helps the dying patients far more than most of us think.

- Patients' psychosocial and spiritual needs are all those things that make us all tick as people.

- Theory helps us to understand people and their behaviour.

- Communicating effectively makes a difference and can be learned.

- There are many things that stop us performing at our best—look out for them.

References

1. Saunders, C. (2006) *Cicely Saunders: Selected Writings 1958–2004*. Oxford, Oxford University Press.
2. Francis R. (2013) *Report of the Mid Staffordshire NHS Foundation Trust Public Inquiry—Executive Summary*. London, The Stationery Office.
3. Parliamentary and Health Service Ombudsman. (2011) *Care and Compassion? Report of the Health Service Ombudsman on Ten Investigations into NHS Care of Older People*. London, The Stationery Office.
4. Gold Standards Framework Centre. (2008) *The PEPSI COLA Aide-memoire*. Available online at <http://www.goldstandardsframework.org.uk/cd-content/uploads/files/Library,%20Tools%20%26%20resources/PepsicolaHPAguidancedocument.pdf>
5. Department of Health. (2011) *Spiritual Care at the End of Life: A Systematic Review of the Literature*. Available online at <https://www.gov.uk/government/uploads/system/uploads/attachment_data/file/215798/dh_123804.pdf> (accessed 30/1/2014)
6. Saunders, C.M. (1967) *The Management of Terminal Illness*. London, Hospital Medicine Publications.
7. Kubler-Ross, E. (1969) *On Death and Dying*. New York, Macmillan.
8. Corr, C.A. (1992) A task-based approach to coping with dying. *Omega*; **24**(2):81–4.
9. Glaser, B.G. and Strauss, A.L. (1965) *Awareness of Dying*. Chicago, Adeline.
10. Timmermans, S. (1994) Dying awareness: the theory of awareness revisited. *Social Health and Illness*; **16**:322–37.
11. Balint, M. (1963) *The Doctor, His Patient and the Illness* (2nd edn). London, Churchill.
12. Heaven, C.M. and Maguire, P. (1996) Training hospice nurses to elicit patient concerns. *Journal of Advanced Nursing*; **23**(2):280–86.

13. **Wilkinson, S., Perry, R., Blanchard, K., et al.** (2008) Effectiveness of a three-day communication skills course in changing nurses' communication skills with cancer/palliative care patients: a randomised trial. *Palliative Medicine*; **22**(4):365–75.

14. **Fallowfield, L., Jenkins, V., Saul, J., et al.** (2002) Efficacy of a cancer research UK communication skills training model for oncologists: a randomised controlled trial. Lancet; **359**(9307):650–56.

15. **Cotton H.** (2013) Framework for a Support network (Unpublished). Available from Cotton H. Personal Communication. Executive Coaching and Leadership. <http://www.not-there-yet.co.uk>

Further reading

Lloyd-Williams, M. (2008) *Psychosocial Issues in Palliative Care* (2nd edn), Oxford, Oxford University Press.

Machin, L. (2009) *Working with Loss and Grief.* London, Sage.

Vachon, M.L.S. (2010) The emotional problems of the patient in palliative medicine. In Hanks, G., Cherny, N.I., Christakis, N.A., et al. (eds). *The Oxford Textbook of Palliative Medicine* (4th edn). Oxford, Oxford University Press.

Decisions and care around the end of life

Decisions and care around the end of life

Death is a universal certainty

Providing treatment and care towards the end of life will often involve decisions that are clinically complex and emotionally distressing; and some decisions may involve ethical dilemmas and uncertainties about the law that further complicate the decision-making process.[1]

Reproduced with permission from General Medical Council, *Treatment and care towards the end of life: good practice in decision making*, GMC, London, UK. Copyright © 2010

There is nothing more certain than all our patients, indeed all of us, will die one day, but unfortunately, even for patients with advanced progressive illness, the circumstances of death happen most often by default rather than by design. It seems that doctors and nurses and other professionals either don't always *recognize* when a patient is nearing the end of his or her life or, maybe, don't *acknowledge* this themselves and share the information with the patient and the family. Caring for sick people who are deteriorating and at risk of dying is most commonly a balance of approaches (Figure 4.1), of hoping and striving for the best but preparing also for the worst.

Maybe it's our training, the culture of health care, or possibly what we are more comfortable with that leads us to focus on the immediate problems caused by the illness and its threat to life. It can be very hard to resist the emphasis on 'doing something' (trying to cure) even when this is just not possible. The 'Learning Exercise' in this section may help you to think about your own values and behaviours.

We sometimes (but evidence suggests not frequently enough) consider the need to relieve the distress caused by the physical symptoms: 'I'll give Mr Kumar some ibuprofen for the hip pain from his prostate cancer'. But how often do we take an overview of the whole situation; assess what has happened over the past weeks and months; find out what life has been like for the patient and their family; find out their views on how this illness episode should be managed? (See also Chapter 3.) How can we hope to provide patients and their relatives with

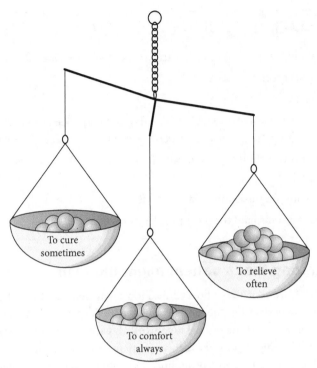

Figure 4.1 The roles of health care professionals: attributed to Hippocrates

the best care at the end of their lives without recognizing and acknowledging that the patient is dying from his or her illness? Think about what Maya Angelou said:

> As a nurse, we have the opportunity to heal the heart, mind, soul and body of our patients, their families and ourselves. They may forget your name, but they will never forget how you made them feel. [2]

? THINK POINTS

- ♦ The quality of care given to dying patients and communication with their relatives is one of the most common causes of complaint.
- ♦ Receiving a complaint is one of the most devastating experiences for professionals.
- ♦ If you and your team don't consider that a patient may be dying, how will you provide them with the best care?

LEARNING EXERCISE

Think about the duties for health care professionals described in Figure 4.1.

- Do you agree?
- Do you *really* agree?
- Do you behave like this in your everyday care for patients? Reflect on care for the last patient you looked after who had very advanced disease.
- How do you think your education has balanced these tenets of health care so far?
- What are you most and least able to do?
- What do you spend the most time learning and practicing?

Recognizing that a patient might die soon

In Chapter 1, we considered how clinical tools may help identify patients who may be at risk of deteriorating and dying. As patients get less well, the concept of *uncertain recovery* is helpful in supporting those who might be very close to dying but who might possibly recover; patients who we really can't be sure about. This dilemma is most pronounced in patients with non-malignant illness where episodic, life-threatening deterioration is part of the 'normal' progressive disease trajectory (e.g. advanced heart failure and chronic obstructive airways disease). *Uncertain recovery* is a way of thinking about what else needs to be done for patients and families as well as trying the best to help a patient recover. The care of such patients is outlined in Box 4.1. For patients who have deteriorated to the point where recovery from an acute or sub-acute illness seems very uncertain, the justification for continuing invasive treatments or monitoring should be reviewed and discussed with patients and carers and between and within professional teams.

Recognizing the onset of dying

There is little evidence to help us reliably spot when a patient may in fact be dying. The following signs are thought to be helpful as indicators:

- Profound weakness
- Gaunt appearance
- Drowsiness
- Disorientation
- Diminished oral intake

Box 4.1 The care of sick patients with *uncertain recovery*

Discussions with the patient (and family)

- Share the uncertainty of prognosis (see 'Handling challenging situations' in Chapter 2).
- Establish patient's and family's concerns and the level of information they would prefer.
- Seek information about patient's preferences and wishes including where they would like to be cared for if they are dying.

Decision making

- Does the patient have capacity to make decisions about their treatment?
- Is there an advance decision to refuse treatment (ADRT)?
- Has a lasting power of attorney (LPA) for health and welfare been appointed?
- Escalation of medical treatments (e.g. intensive care/non-invasive ventilation/dialysis)
- Resuscitation status

Care plan

- Physical symptom management
- Spiritual care needs
- Clear documentation of patient's wishes and clinical decisions

- Difficulty taking oral medication
- Poor concentration
- Skin colour changes (pale or blue)
- Temperature change at extremities (cold nose and hands)

Probably the most important element in recognizing or diagnosing dying is that the members of the multi-professional team caring for the patient agree that the patient is likely to die. Where there is disagreement between team members, there are opposing goals of care, and then mixed messages are presented to the patient and their family. Barriers to recognizing that this is the situation for the patient and making appropriate decisions for their care decisions are shown in Box 4.2.

Box 4.2 Barriers to 'diagnosing dying'[3]

♦ Hope that the patient may get better

♦ No definitive disease diagnosis: no one sure why this is happening

♦ Pursuance of unrealistic or futile interventions

♦ Disagreement in the team about the patient's condition

♦ Failure to recognize key symptoms and signs

♦ Poor ability to communicate with the family and patient

♦ Concerns about withdrawing or withholding treatment

♦ Fear of foreshortening life

♦ Concerns about resuscitation

♦ Cultural and spiritual barriers

♦ Medico-legal concerns

Reproduced from Ellershaw, J.E. and Ward, C., 'Care of the dying Patient: the last hours or days of life', *British Medical Journal*, Volume 326, Number 7379, pp. 30–34, Copyright © 2003, with permission from BMJ Publishing Group.

A good death needs good decisions: what are the 'right' decisions for patients?

Decision making with patients with advanced progressive illnesses who may be dying is complex. It is seldom black and white. We must decide what to do and what not to do. We must resist the urge to undertake a medical intervention without some evidence that it will be of help to the patient. We must weigh up the benefits and the harms or adverse effects. In a situation which is often sad and, of course, unwanted, we need to think through the question: *What seems most right for this patient*? Guidance from the General Medical Council[1] is really helpful and it is important to take time to read it if you are a doctor or medical student.

Our decisions are helped by applying our knowledge of medical ethics to the patient's situation (Box 4.3). In reading this chapter, you should call to mind these ethical 'pillars' of clinical judgement.

The 'Case History Exercise' in this section will help you to think about these issues and how you make decisions with patients, their families, and the health care team.

Box 4.3 Medical ethics in decision making in advanced disease

Decision making is underpinned by the principles or 'pillars' of medical ethics:

- ◆ beneficence
- ◆ non-maleficence
- ◆ justice
- ◆ respect for autonomy

If you haven't yet explored medical ethics, a good place to start is *Ethical Issues in Palliative Care*. [4]

 CASE HISTORY EXERCISE

You have been called to see Mrs Collins at home, who has severe Parkinson's disease. You've seen her three or four times this year. She has become progressively immobile and her husband tells you that she has been in bed for the past two weeks. You have been called because she has a painful and disturbing cough. You think it likely that she has pneumonia. She is hypoxic, tachycardic, and hypotensive. You think she may die. You tell her she needs to be in hospital and her head 'goes down'. 'Do I have any choice?' she asks.

How will you take this further to make the best plan for Mrs Collins? What are the things you will need to discuss with her and her husband? Write short notes on the options for management of this lady. Think how the four ethical principles are at play here and how they will influence your decision. (See our thoughts in 'Case history exercise: some thoughts on Mrs Collins' in this chapter.)

Patient autonomy: it is the patient's decision, not ours

The patient's view on how their illness, life, and death should be managed is vital, and their autonomy in this is generally of key ethical importance. In a patient who is able to talk to you and is competent, this relies on you communicating well with them and providing them with high-quality information about the natural history of the condition and the likely benefits and potential problems of the treatments you are proposing. You need to inform patients accurately of their choices, in order for them to make decisions. Their choice is what counts, even if it differs from the choice of their family, our 'advice', or what may be considered 'normal'. Some patients would prefer, however, to let others in their family make the decision or make the decision as a family together. That's their choice.

Decision making is more complex when a patient is unconscious, confused, or lacking capacity for other reasons. Box 4.4 tells you more about decision making and mental capacity. When a patient lacks capacity for the decision, as

---

Box 4.4 Does the patient have the capacity to make this decision?

The Mental Capacity Act in England and Wales[5] sets out the criteria to assess whether a patient has the capacity to make a decision. It is important to remember that capacity is decision specific and that the same patient may have capacity to make decisions for some things (e.g. coffee or tea) but not others. A patient is judged competent to make a decision when they are able to:

♦ comprehend the information relevant to the decision (which requires the information to have been presented to that person in a way appropriate to their circumstances);

♦ retain this information for long enough to make the decision;

♦ use and weigh the information to arrive at a choice (which requires an understanding of the consequences of making a decision one way or the other);

♦ communicate the decision (which requires enablement, e.g. with an interpreter or speech aid).

The following may make the patient lack capacity to make a decision:

♦ reduced conscious state from injury, drugs, or infection

♦ disorientation from mental illness

♦ cerebral diseases, e.g. Alzheimer's

♦ congenital mental disability

♦ locked-in syndrome

♦ coercion from others

Reproduced from *Mental Capacity Act 2005*, © Crown Copyright, licensed under the Open Government License v.2.0, available at <http://www.legislation.gov.uk/ukpga/2005/9/contents>

far as possible decisions should still be based on their known wishes. Their autonomy is still of prime ethical importance when making decisions in their best interest.

Best interest decision

When a patient lacks capacity for a decision, it is the responsibility of the senior clinician involved with the patient to make that decision. The clinician must consider:

- the person's past and present wishes and feelings (including written advance statements);
- any beliefs and values (for example, religious, cultural, or moral) that would be likely to influence the decision in question;
- any other relevant factors.

The GMC guidance states that the decisions you or others make on the patient's behalf must be based on whether treatment would be of overall benefit to the patient, and which option (including the option not to treat) would be least restrictive of the patient's future choices. As far as possible, the decision maker must consult other people and take into account their views as to what would be in the best interests of the person lacking capacity, especially:

- anyone previously named by the person lacking capacity as someone to be consulted;
- carers, close relatives or close friends, or anyone else interested in the person's welfare.

Planning care in advance and advance statements about treatments

There is growing evidence that discussions about what may happen and making a potential plan for care in line with the patient's wishes can improve the quality of life of patients with advanced disease[6] and increase carer satisfaction.[7,8] The process of care planning aims to promote shared decision making through voluntary dialogue between health care professionals and the patient, relative, or nominated other (if the patient lacks capacity to make decisions) about their care.

Discussions incorporating relevant medical information and individual preferences can help determine a care plan that outlines proposed appropriate actions for specific clinical situations that might arise in the course of the patient's illness. Such an emergency health care plan provides useful information to share across teams (nursing, medical, etc.) and services (hospital, GP, out of hours, etc.) so that everyone knows what the patient would most like to happen and how they would like to be cared for. These discussions also help patients and relatives know what might happen and be a little more prepared to make decisions when things do change. So, for example, if a patient with terminal cardiopulmonary disease (COPD) has distressing breathlessness, they may call the community nursing service rather than 999, so that they continue to be cared for at home.

Some patients may make their own written record of their wishes with respect to medical interventions, especially those they wish to refuse. Some patients may also appoint a family member or friend as an Lasting Power of Attorney LPA for making decisions regarding health and welfare, if they lose capacity.

Advance statements and care plans guide health care professionals when those circumstances arise and the patient does not have the capacity to make the decision with the clinician. Advance statements can have:

+ a statement of general beliefs and values;
+ a requesting statement reflecting the individual's aspirations and preferences;
+ a clear instruction refusing some or all medical procedures (advance decision to refuse treatment: ADRT);
+ a statement that specifies a degree of irreversible impairment after which no life-sustaining treatment should be given;
+ a statement that names a person who should be consulted about decisions.

Most of these statements are a guide to clinicians, a suggested emergency health care plan made when there was time to talk and think before the crisis arose. However, ADRTs and LPA have legal force if they are made by a competent patient, are constructed in the required way, and are applicable to the specific circumstances that have arisen. Advance statements which request clinical treatments which are at odds with clinical judgement about the patient's best interests, do not have legal force.

In our experience, although some patients do write advance statements, many find that this is emotionally too difficult to do themselves. Some may be able to construct a plan together with a health professional who is usually, but not exclusively, their doctor. These sort of discussions and plans are normally done in stages and the piecemeal recording of discussions with patients, concerning their general and specific views, is important in helping the clinical team, and especially the palliative care team, to make the best decisions if circumstances mean that the patient is unable to guide us.

The 'Learning Exercise' that follows may help you apply this knowledge to real-life clinical work.

LEARNING EXERCISE

When you next see a patient with a major stroke who can't communicate, think about:

◆ How do you know what decisions the patient would make about the treatments you or the health care team think are and are not clinically appropriate?

◆ What are you basing these judgements on?

◆ How do you find out what the patient's wishes would be?

Then ask members of the team who are looking after the patient what their thoughts are and how they made decisions.

If you want to know more about advance care planning and emergency health care plans look at <http://www.cnne.org.uk/end-of-life-care—the-clinical-network/decidingright>

I want to die: requests for euthanasia or help with suicide

If you listen to patients who have very advanced illness, it isn't unusual that they will tell you that they want to die. A few will ask you to end it for them. How are you going to handle this?

In the UK, both euthanasia and help from a health professional to commit suicide are illegal. But a request to die demands more than simply a 'no-can-do' type response. It is clearly a very serious matter. It is often a sign of great distress, usually both physical and emotional. It is also a sign that they feel they can trust you. Chapter 2 discusses the development of your communication skills in handling this situation.

In our experience, many patients feel this distressed from time to time. Living with advanced illness and the prospect of getting worse and dying is not easy. However, most do not actually want euthanasia. It is only when they trust you enough to listen, without judgement, fear, or avoidance, that they can share their distress of having to carry on living like this. For many patients, the intensity of this feeling varies from day to day. The reasons that may lie behind a request to die include:

◆ poorly controlled symptoms;

◆ fears: about dying, being a burden, things getting intolerable;

+ depression;
+ feeling overwhelmed and unable to cope;
+ loss of control/need for control.

Many of these issues can at least be alleviated for most patients, often with help from a specialist palliative care team. It is also vital to never underestimate the therapeutic impact you can have by listening. You may not be able to change much about the patient's situation but allowing them to express their distress and talk *can* lighten the degree of it.

? THINK POINT

One study in a hospice service in The Netherlands (where euthanasia is legal) has analysed the context of people's requests for euthanasia. Twenty to 30% of patients requested euthanasia at some point; 1.6% of patients actually left the hospice for euthanasia.

Euthanasia and assisted suicide are complex ethical, moral, and legal issues. To do them justice is beyond the scope of this text, and further reading is indicated at the end of the chapter.

? THINK POINT

We cannot judge, as external observers, the circumstances which make suffering intolerable to any one individual. The young, bed-bound woman with every tube imaginable in place, with whom I sat and watched *EastEnders* as Ethel asked Dot to help her die, told me she believed strongly in euthanasia, that we don't let dogs suffer like we do humans. 'Are you suffering?' I asked, expecting a very tricky conversation. 'Oh no. Life's OK' she said, to my amazement.

Deciding when to stop life-sustaining treatments and when not to start them

For people with advanced incurable progressive illness, the focus of their care is based on the quality of their lives. As their health deteriorates, it might be that particular treatments or interventions are considered, such as antibiotics for life- threatening infection, cardiopulmonary resuscitation (CPR), renal dialysis, artificial nutrition and hydration, and mechanical ventilation.

The health care team must weigh up carefully the appropriateness of use of treatments. The three key considerations are:

- Will they enhance the quality of life?
- Do the benefits outweigh the burdens?
- Are they certain not to lengthen suffering or the dying process?

The evidence of the benefits, burdens, and risks of treatments is not always clear cut, and there may be uncertainty about the clinical effect of a treatment on an individual patient or about the particular benefits, burdens, and risks for that patient. All such decisions must be considered in a holistic context. For instance, will interventions possibly stop the patient going home?

Taking everything into account, the doctor must first identify which investigations or treatments are clinically appropriate and likely to result in overall benefit for the patient. These options are then discussed with the patient, setting out the potential benefits, burdens, and risks of each option and the uncertainties. A patient with capacity may have clear views on what potential treatments they do and don't want. Only patients themselves can judge the quality of their lives (see previous 'Think Point'). The doctor may recommend a particular option which they believe to be best for the patient, but they must not pressure the patient to accept their advice.

For very sick patients who are not able to communicate their views on treatments and interventions, and for those who lack capacity for other reasons, a framework for decision making is important (Figure 4.2). In these circumstances, unless the patient has appointed an LPA, it is the doctor who will have to make the best interest decisions for the patient, based on 'overall benefit'.

In the dying patient, hydration and nutrition are common issues of concern to relatives and professionals. If a patient wants to drink, then they should be helped to do so. Table 4.1 indicates some of the considerations necessary in making the decision about the administration of parenteral fluids to a dying patient. Many patients, dying from their very advanced illness, do not feel like eating and artificial nutrition is usually clinically inappropriate. It's important to help the family understand that the patient's body cannot utilize nutrition at this point and that it will do more harm than good.

The previous 'Learning Exercise' may help you think about the challenges and importance of making decisions about care for very sick patients.

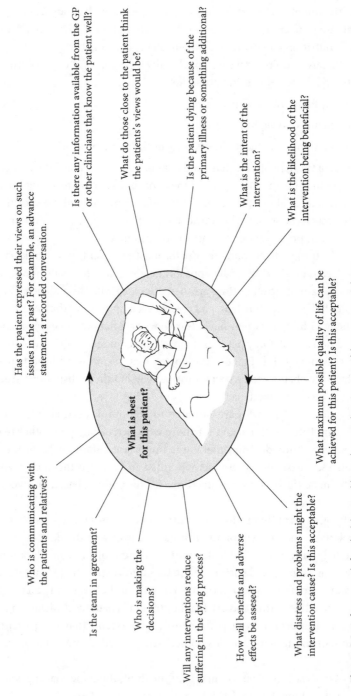

Figure 4.2 A framework for decision making when patients are unable to communicate their views about treatments

Is there any information available from the GP or other clinicians that know the patient well?

What do those close to the patient think the patients's views would be?

Is the patient dying because of the primary illness or something additional?

What is the intent of the intervention?

What is the likelihood of the intervention being beneficial?

Has the patient expressed their views on such issues in the past? For example, an advance statement, a recorded conversation.

What is best for this patient?

What maximun possible quality of life can be achieved for this patient? Is this acceptable?

What distress and problems might the intervention cause? Is this acceptable?

How will benefits and adverse effects be assesed?

Will any interventions reduce suffering in the dying process?

Who is making the decisions?

Is the team in agreement?

Who is communicating with the patients and relatives?

Table 4.1 Artificial hydration (IV/SC fluids) during the dying phase: to use or not to use?

PROS	CONS
May reduce thirst in some patients (but good mouth care usually does as good a job).	May stop patients being at home.
Seems less like we're just letting the patient die (but remember, he or she is dying from the disease, not dehydration). (Ask: who are we treating really—us, the relatives, or the patient?)	May make death less 'natural', i.e. medicalized. Families may be less able to cuddle and get close with the pump/drip stand and infusion set getting in the way.
May help circulation of drugs to relieve symptoms.	May make nurses less likely to give good mouth care.
May reduce confusion.	May cause pulmonary oedema.
	May increase incontinence/restlessness from full bladder.
	Venflons are painful and infusion sets constraining.

 CASE HISTORY EXERCISE

Mrs Pierce has had multiple sclerosis for 25 years. She has been admitted with pneumonia. She is unable to communicate and she cannot protect her airway when swallowing. You recognize that she may be dying. You need to consider whether you are going to:

♦ give her antibiotics;

♦ put up a drip;

♦ organize enteral feeding;

♦ attempt CPR;

♦ get her home.

Think about how you might make these decisions. If you have a chance, discuss your thoughts with a doctor or senior nurse.

(See our thoughts in 'Case history exercise: some thoughts on Mrs Pierce' in this chapter.)

Cardiopulmonary resuscitation

Cardiopulmonary resuscitation (CPR) can be attempted on any individual in whom cardiac or respiratory function ceases. Of course, the stopping of breathing and of the heart happens as part of dying, and although CPR could theoretically be used on every individual who dies, this would seem inappropriate and deny the normality and certainty of death. Making and recording an advance decision *do not attempt CPR* (DNA-CPR) will help to ensure that the patient dies in a dignified and peaceful manner and allow their family to be with them. It may also help to ensure that the patient's last hours or days are spent in their preferred place of care by, for example, avoiding emergency admission from a community setting to hospital.

The key issues in considering whether resuscitation is appropriate for a patient with an advanced progressive disease are:

◆ Does cessation of cardiac and respiratory function represent the terminal event of that illness, i.e. have they 'died' rather than 'arrested'?

◆ Is CPR likely to be effective?

◆ What are the burdens and benefits of CPR, what quality of life would CPR regain and what are the patient's views on this?

◆ Does this patient want to be resuscitated if the treatment was thought to be effective? (In our experiences, many with advanced diseases do not want this, but some do.)

Guidance on decision making is available (Box 4.5). Your organization will have its own policy which you should be familiar with. If resuscitation is not to be undertaken, a DNA-CPR form needs to be completed and the form should be kept with the patient, when at home, and in the ward or care home files.

 LEARNING EXERCISE

In one study, nearly 50% of hospice in-patients with advanced cancer said they would definitely wish to be resuscitated if their heart stopped suddenly. Patients, however, vastly overestimate the success of resuscitation. What is the success rate of CPR in advanced cancer? How do we share this information?

Look at the reference in the 'Cardiopulmonary resuscitation' section of 'Further reading and resources' at the end of this chapter. Work through the e-ELCA session 03–30 'Discussing "do not attempt CPR" decisions'.

It is recommended best practice to always discuss the decision with the patient and the family. In some circumstances, you are informing the patient and family about a DNA-CPR decision; in other circumstances, you are seeking their views and sharing a decision with the patient. The approaches to these two situations are different.

Box 4.5 BMA, RCN, and Resuscitation Council guidelines[9]

It is appropriate to consider a do not attempt CPR (DNA-CPR) decision in the following circumstances:

- If the healthcare team is as certain as it can be that a person is dying as an inevitable result of underlying disease or a catastrophic health event, and CPR would not re-start the heart and breathing

- Where the patient's condition indicates that CPR is unlikely to be successful.

- Where CPR is not in accord with the sustained wishes of the patient who is mentally competent.

- Where a patient, lacking capacity, has a valid and applicable advance decision refusing treatment (ADRT), specifically refusing CPR,.

- Where successful CPR is likely to be followed by a length and quality of life which would not be in the best interests of a patient who lacks capacity.

Source: data from *Decisions Relating to Cardiopulmonary Resuscitation: A Joint Statement from the British Medical Association, the Resuscitation Council (UK), and the Royal College of Nursing*, Copyright © British Medical Association 2014

Informing, not asking

If CPR is not likely to be effective, and a DNA-CPR decision has been made for that reason, then this information needs to be shared sensitively with the patient and the family. It is important not to ask what they want, since there is no choice; CPR will not work. It is very important, however, to elicit their concerns and questions about the decision. People generally have a lot of misunderstandings about the success and the level of trauma of resuscitation. Usually, it is helpful to discuss the heart stopping in the context of an end-of-life care plan and in relation to how the DNA-CPR form is important to help achieve what the patient and family want. Box 4.6 gives an example of a conversation with a patient about a DNA-CPR decision.

It's thought good practice to discuss the DNA-CPR decision with the patient, unless you think that this will cause physical or psychological harm. You shouldn't avoid discussing it because it's uncomfortable for you. For many patients who are dying, however, there may be more important things to discuss and it is essential not to burden them with long conversations. Extremely sick patients are very

---

Box 4.6 Informing, not asking

A heart failure specialist nurse discusses the resuscitation decision with Mr Smith who has advanced heart failure

Having discussed with Mr Smith his understanding of his illness, and gained some idea of what's important to him in the future, the nurse now begins to negotiate actions that will support Mr Smith's wishes and develop an antici-patory emergency health care plan.

Mr Smith, thank you for sharing your thoughts about what you think is hap-pening. It's really helpful to know that it's important for you to be at home if things worsen and be cared for by the family as much as possible.

One of the things that is useful to make sure this can happen is for me to leave certain forms in the house so that should you need to call anyone in an emer-gency, they know what we have discussed and what the plan is. One of the things that people want to know in an emergency is what to do about resuscita-tion, if your heart or breathing were to stop. Unfortunately, your heart isn't going to respond to that treatment. As you've already shared with me, staying at home and having your family with you right to the end is what you'd prefer. With that in mind, I would like to complete and leave in your home, the DNA-CPR paperwork that will allow that to happen. If an ambulance is called, they will know to try and keep you comfortable, but won't try to take you to hospital or revive you.

Are there things about that which you would like to discuss further?

---

fatigued and there are usually more significant things (from their perspective) for them to be spending valuable time on. They will want to be with the impor-tant people in their lives, not intruded upon unduly by the health care team. If the decision is not discussed you will need to record, in the notes, your reasons for not discussing the decision with the patient.

Seeing a DNA-CPR form, which hasn't been discussed, can cause patients and family great distress and anxiety. If the form is to be in the patient's home, they need to know about it and have the opportunity to voice concerns and ask questions.

Asking: shared decision making

When resuscitation has a reasonable chance of working, we usually need to discuss the patient's views on what they would choose. This may be because they might not want life to be prolonged should their arrest be 'out of the blue' or because they would not want to live with a worse quality of life (a common consequence of a cardiac arrest and resuscitation).

Research indicates that even though discussing these decisions is complex and worrying, more patients would like to be involved in these discussions than we currently approach. The following 'Learning Exercise' may help you apply this thinking and guidance.

 LEARNING EXERCISE

- Observe the process of making the DNA-CPR decision with the next patient with an advanced, life-threatening illness you are involved with.
- Go with your medical team when they discuss CPR status with a patient and relatives.
- How are the nurses involved in the decision?
- How is the decision recorded?
- Speak to the doctors and nurses about how they discuss these issues with the patient and the family.
- Be aware that many teams do not always follow best practice. So, if you see a decision made that does not follow the guidance, that does not mean they have done it correctly!

How can you help people die in the place of their choice?

Most people say they would, ideally, wish to die at home. Theoretically, this should be achievable for those who die from progressive diseases, but it only happens for about one person in four. One of the key things that needs to happen is for professionals to talk with patients about their concerns and wishes. Figure 4.3 illustrates some common scenarios that can arise for patients and their families and the barriers that lead to people not dying in the place that they would ideally like to.

When it comes to it, not everyone will choose to die at home, but the research on what may prevent this happening has implications for the way you can best work with patients and their families to help them achieve the best possible outcome in their particular circumstances. It may be that they need information or practical help. It may be that they need to discuss with someone their perspectives and worries as a family. Figure 4.4 illustrates the work they need you to do to help them achieve the best possible outcome.

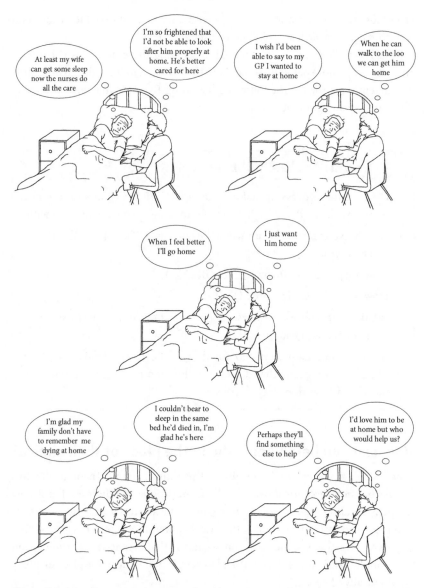

Figure 4.3 Missed opportunity: some thoughts, miscommunications, misunderstandings, and circumstances that can lead to patients not dying at home

Care in the last days of life

When a patient is recognized as dying, it is important that the clinical team have a clear, individualized care plan to ensure that the patient's and their family's needs are fully assessed, that communication is effective and frequent, and that problems and symptoms are managed well. At the time of writing, there is much

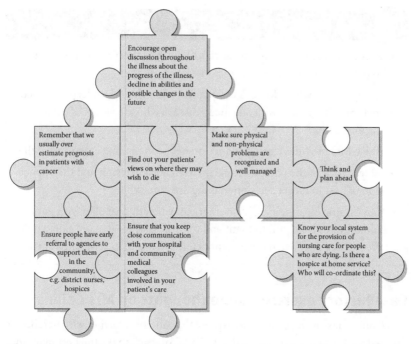

Figure 4.4 The fundamental pieces of the work you will need to do to enable people to die in the place of their choice

focus on this area of care in the NHS in England and Wales and new NICE guidance on end of life care is expected in 2016.

👁 **SUMMARY BOX**

Decision making with and about people who are dying is complex. We have immense power, as professionals, which we have to use wisely to facilitate the best possible choices, decisions, and outcomes for patients. The ethical principles of autonomy, non-maleficence, beneficence, and justice underpin such decision making alongside the need for compassion, good communication, team working, and a sound knowledge of the benefits and harms of treatments and interventions and medico-legal and local clinical governance policies.

Everybody dies. The aim is to make it as good as possible for every individual. Finding out what this might mean for each person, recording their wishes, and acting accordingly, are vital components of helping patients achieve what they most desire.

KEY POINTS

- Recognizing that patients are at risk of deterioration and dying is crucial to patient outcomes.
- An approach which focuses on quality of life should underpin decision making with people with advanced disease who are at risk of deteriorating and dying.
- The GMC provides clear guidance on decision making at the end of life.
- Assessment of the patient's capacity to make a decision and the application of best interests decision making are core skills.
- Developing an anticipatory or emergency health care plan with patients and families is helpful to them and to professionals that are called on to provide support when the patient deteriorates and in crisis situations.

Case history exercise: some thoughts on Mrs Collins

Mrs Collins has given you a cue to explore this situation further with her. Before discussing the choices, open the discussion. You can't make the best plan until you understand all the components that should be considered. You will need to try and find out:

- What is she concerned about? Is she concerned about being admitted to hospital, wanting to stay at home, not wanting active treatment, or something else? (It may well be something you can't guess at and you need to ask. Remember, we shouldn't make assumptions—we may be wrong!)
- What are her thoughts about her life and her illness in general?
- What are her thoughts about her future care?
- Have you explained to her fully enough what you think is happening?
- Has she understood what you have discussed?
- Are there questions she wants to ask you?

The choices

There are four possible plans:

1. To admit to hospital for intensive treatment. Would she/you consider ventilation as appropriate if it is clinically indicated?
2. To admit to a GP unit/cottage hospital/care home (if available). Is this to provide the nursing care or the medical treatments she needs? Does she need an X-ray, blood gases, or other hospital-type support?

3. To stay at home with extra nursing care, analgesia, oxygen, and antibiotics, started intravenously (IV) and then continued orally. Can you organize this tonight? Can you get a physiotherapist tomorrow? Can you review tomorrow? This will provide good palliation, but if the intent is to cure her, then the risk is that this will be suboptimal treatment. (Her hypotension suggests she may be septic and would need more intensive observations as she is at risk of deteriorating rapidly.)

4. To stay at home. Manage the pain with a small dose of morphine and review tomorrow. The intent here is to palliate symptoms but not prolong life.

Case history exercise: some thoughts on Mrs Pierce

To help us make the best decisions for Mrs Pierce, we need to know as much as possible about her.

◆ Before this pneumonia, what was she able to do?

◆ What has the quality of her life been like in the past couple of months?

◆ Has she made any written advance statements or had conversations with those close to her?

◆ Has she appointed an LPA for health and welfare?

◆ Do her relatives or friends know what her thoughts would be in her current situation?

◆ Does she appear distressed by physical things; pain, cough, breathing?

◆ Does she appear emotionally distressed; is she restless, clasping your hand, frowning? (She may, of course, not have the motor function to do any of these things.)

Remember that putting IV lines in and inserting nasogastric tubes have associated risks and discomfort. If the patient is dying, it can make the process clinical and not allow the relatives to be close. Drip stands and infusion lines can form an actual and indirect barrier around a patient. You must be sure that there are benefits to gain. You will need to keep this under review, as your approach may change over the next few days.

Unless she is able to cough, it is unlikely that her pneumonia will be cured by antibiotics alone. You need to make a decision about how 'active' you are going to be. Do you need further investigations to aid you in this (e.g. X-ray, blood gases, blood cultures)? Are they going to affect your management plan? Don't do them for the sake of it. Would ventilation be appropriate? You will need to discuss this with your senior doctor. The decision about her resuscitation status must also be documented. Antibiotics may, however, reduce the quantity of sputum, if this is distressing to her. If you decide to start them, you should review their benefit after 24 hours.

Mrs Pierce is unlikely to be distressed by thirst if good mouth care is undertaken by the nursing staff. In addition, fluid administration may cause pulmonary oedema. If your management plan is one of intensive treatment with a view to recovery, then fluids should be used with caution and their benefits and adverse effects reviewed daily. If she gets worse, then you should plan to withdraw them. It's helpful to discuss this with the patient and family as you start them, so that they know that you will review things and might decide to stop them.

Assisted nutrition (enteral feeding) is not clinically appropriate in the acute stage of her illness. However, the relatives may be concerned about it and you should discuss the fact that she does not need it immediately, that she is not hungry or suffering without it, and that it carries some risks while she is so ill. If she improves, this will of course need to be reviewed and patients should always be offered food to see if they desire it.

 SUMMARY BOX

Ethical and legal considerations

What does she want?	Autonomy
Are you doing any good?	Beneficence
Are you doing any harm?	Non-maleficence
Is the intervention the best use of resources?	Justice
Are you obeying the law?	Legality

References

1. **General Medical Council.** (2010) *Treatment and care towards the end of life: good practice in decision making.* London, GMC. <http://www.gmc-uk.org/guidance/ethical_guidance/end_of_life_guidance.asp>

2. **Angelou, M.** (2014) Inspirational Nursing Quotes, Nursing Licence Map. Available from <http://nursinglicensemap.com/nursing-quotes/>

3. **Ellershaw, J.E. and Ward, C.** (2003) Care of the dying patient: the last hours or days of life . *BMJ*; **326**:30–34.

4. **De Caestecker, S.** (2012) Ethical issues in palliative care. In Faull, C., De Caestecker, S., Nicholson, A., Black, F. (eds) *Handbook of Palliative Care* (3rd edn). New Jersey, Wiley-Blackwell.

5. **Mental Capacity Act 2005.** Available at <http://www.legislation.gov.uk/ukpga/2005/9/contents>

6. **Wright, A.A., Zhang, B., Ray, A., et al.** (2008) Associations between end-of-life discussions, patient mental health, medical care near death, and caregiver bereavement adjustment. *JAMA*; **300**:1665–73.

7. **Detering, K.M., Hancock, A.D., Reade, M.C., and Silvester, W.** (2010) The impact of advance care planning on end of life care in elderly patients: randomised controlled trial. *BMJ*; **340**: c1345.

8. **Teno, J.M., Gruneir, A., Schwartz, Z., Nanda, A., and Wetle, T.** (2007) Association between advance directives and quality of end-of-life care: a national study. *J Am Geriatr Soc*; **55**:189–94.

9. **British Medical Association.** (2014) Decisions Relating to Cardiopulmonary Resuscitation. A Joint Statement from the British Medical Association, the Resuscitation Council (UK), and the Royal College of Nursing. <https://www.resus.org.uk/pages/DecisionsRelatingToCPR.pdf>

Further reading and resources

Ethics and ethical dilemmas

Gillon, R. (1994) Medical ethics: four principles plus attention to scope. *BMJ*; **309**:184–8.

Randall, F. and Downie, R.S. (1999) *Palliative Care Ethics: A Companion for Specialists* (2nd edn). Oxford, Oxford University Press.

Roy, D.J. and MacDonald, N. (1998) Ethical issues in palliative care. In Doyle, D., Hanks, G.W.C., and MacDonald N. (eds). *Oxford Textbook of Palliative Medicine*. Oxford, Oxford University Press.

Advance care planning

Mullick, A., Martin, J., and Sallnow, L. (2013) An introduction to advance care planning in practice. *BMJ*; **347**:f6064.

NHS North East. Deciding right: resources for supporting advance care planning. <http://www.cnne.org.uk/end-of-life-care—the-clinical-network/decidingright>

Seymour, J., Almack, K., and Kennedy, S. (2010) Implementing advance care planning: a qualitative study of community nurses' views and experiences. *BMC Palliative Care*; **9**:4.

Cardiopulmonary resuscitation

NHS National End of Life Care Programme. (2012) DNACPR decisions: who decides and how? Available at <http://www.nhsiq.nhs.uk/media/2395952/dnacpr_web_resource_final_27.09.12:pdf>

Fisher J. (2010). e-ELCA session 03_30, Discussing 'do not attempt CPR decisions' NHS Health Education England. Available at <http://www.e-lfh.org.uk/projects/end-of-life-care/>

CHAPTER 5

Physical symptom control: how to do it well

Physical symptom control: how to do it well

Introduction to physical symptom control

The aim of this chapter is to help you feel equipped to be on the front line of managing symptoms and using controlled and other drugs. Most certainly you will need to develop your knowledge and skills in this if you are a medical student or doctor, but nurses and support workers also need understanding of symptoms and management strategies. Some of this will be about you learning how to approach clinical problems, and some will be about gaining knowledge of what drugs and other therapies to use and how to prescribe and use them for best effect. However, some of it is about challenging yourself about your behaviour towards patients with pain, nausea, and distress of other sorts. In addition, providing care for patients in the very last stages of their lives has been found to be a challenge and a duty from which many professionals appear to shrink (Box 5.1).

Box 5.1 Mrs N's story[1]

Mrs N was in severe pain and had probable lung cancer, but was waiting for test results to confirm this. Her unbearable pain brought her to hospital where a pain management plan was drawn up. But it was 5 days before she received adequate pain relief. On one occasion, Mrs N had asked for pain relief, only to be told that she had already taken it. However, when the Macmillan Nurse checked the drugs chart, that was not the case. As her daughter observed, 'our mother continued to suffer for too long'. Mrs N died 2 months later. Mrs N's daughter asked the Ombudsman to investigate, who found that management of Mrs N's pain was neglected. Although a pain management plan was in place, nurses seemed unaware of her specific pain management requirements and did not act in accordance with NMC guidelines.

Adapted with permission from *Care and Compassion? Ten investigations into care of older people*, Parliamentary and Health Service Ombudsman, Copyright © 2011 Parliamentary and Health Service Ombudsman.

This chapter is not comprehensive in its coverage of symptoms and their management, and additional sources of information are listed in 'Further reading' at the end of the chapter. A wide range of drugs is available for symptom management and this can seem daunting. Familiarity and a good working knowledge of a relatively small group, that you may need on a frequent basis, are of prime importance, and these drugs are indicated at the end of the chapter. Only morphine has been explored in any depth in this text and you should use other textbooks to familiarize yourself with the pharmacology of the others, including important side-effects, cautions and interactions, and methods of administration.

What physical symptoms do patients with advanced disease experience?

Several studies have shown a high prevalence of distressing physical problems experienced by patients with advanced disease (malignant and non-malignant) (Table 5.1). Pain is clearly a key symptom, but symptoms such as anorexia and fatigue are often paid little serious attention by professionals even though they have a very high prevalence and may be of great distress to patients and relatives.

 LEARNING EXERCISE

Elicit and list all the physical symptoms that the next three patients with advanced disease that you talk to have, and compare the list with Table 5.1. What additional problems do your patients have?

Table 5.1 The prevalence of symptoms in advanced disease (derived from a variety of patient populations and study methodologies).

Symptom	Cancer (%)	Coronary heart disease (%)	COPD(%)	Advanced renal disease (%)
Pain	70	60	65	50
Trouble breathing	40	50	95	60
Nausea or vomiting	40	45	Not known	30
Fatigue/weakness	70	75	90	76
Depression	30	25	40	40
Anorexia	50	40	Not known	47
Constipation	50	30	40	35
Anxiety	40	45	65	55

Improving outcomes for patients

Although we are well aware that physical symptoms in patients with advanced disease are common, many of these symptoms remain uncontrolled for patients. If we were to use this as a performance indicator, we would be in the third division and being relegated. Why is this? Some symptoms are difficult to manage but, for the majority of patients, a big difference can be made with low-tech, simple interventions requiring quite a small amount of knowledge. Our experience has taught us that the key to achieving best symptom management is the application of principles and rules that underpin our care and incorporate factual knowledge and technical and communication skills.

Like becoming a good driver, you must have some *factual knowledge* about how the car works, what you must do to make it go and function at its best performance, and who to *ask for help* if it breaks down; but to get safely to where you want to go, you must apply the principles and *rules of the highway code* (Figure 5.1).

> **? THINK POINT**
>
> Pain is a problem for more than 50% of patients with advanced diseases (not just cancer).

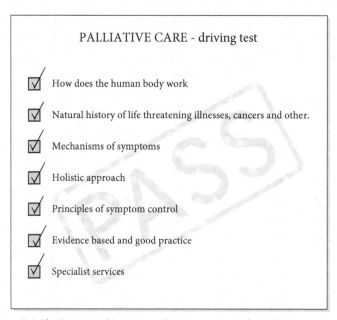

Figure 5.1 The keys to achieving good symptom control can be yours

The principles of good symptom management

Anticipation

It can often be anticipated that an individual patient may run into specific problems and, in some instances, you can prevent the predicted problem occurring. Thinking ahead gives you a better chance of nipping it in the bud, before things require crisis management. Failure to anticipate problems and to set up appropriate management pathways (e.g. who they should call) is a common source of dissatisfaction and preventable suffering for patients.

> **Rule 1: Always think ahead**

 LEARNING EXERCISE

- ◆ What problems should you anticipate might occur when a patient starts taking codeine?
- ◆ What should you do to prevent them?

If you don't know the answers, the 'Management of pain' section later in this chapter should help you.

Understanding of the natural history of the disease with specific reference to an individual patient, awareness of the patient's psychosocial circumstances, and identification of 'risk factors' allow forward planning of care by the health care team.

 CASE HISTORY EXERCISE

Petunia, a 45-year-old married woman with children aged 7 and 11, was recently found to have spinal metastases from her breast cancer.

Write short notes on the potential issues you should anticipate have a high risk of occurring for her in the future. Think about what will need to be discussed and in place to prevent unnecessary suffering and crises, and to optimize symptom control.

Evaluation and assessment

An understanding of the mechanisms and likely cause(s) of any particular problem is fundamental in selecting and directing appropriate investigations and treatment. When asked to see a patient to relieve distress, always, through careful history and examination, try to diagnose the cause of the symptom and decide whether it is possible and appropriate to remove the underlying cause, or at least ameliorate it, in addition to providing concomitant symptomatic relief. For example:

- Abdominal pain due to opioid-related constipation is better treated with suppositories or enemas than with opiates. (Have you seen this vicious circle in action? It is common.)
- Catheterization for an agitated patient with urinary retention is obviously more helpful than sedation.
- Antiemetics for the nausea of hypercalcaemia are important, but so may be lowering the serum calcium.

Be aware. Co-morbidity is common and should *always* be considered. For example, it is easy (and unfortunately common) to assume that pain in a patient with cancer is caused by the cancer. In one case series, almost a quarter of pains in patients with cancer were unrelated to the cancer or the cancer treatment.

Rule 2: Always compile a list of possible causes of symptoms

 LEARNING EXERCISE

Ask the next patient you see who is on regular opioids about his or her bowels. If constipated, ask them how this affects them. How embarrassing is it? Check the laxatives they are prescribed.

The multidimensional nature of symptoms such as pain means that the use of drugs may be only part of a multi-professional team strategy addressing physical, psychological, social, and spiritual distress. A patient's suffering always needs to be understood within its psychosocial context. Only by thinking holistically will we recognize those aspects of the patient's care that need approaches other than the use of drugs. For instance, the concept of total pain (see Chapter 3) acknowledges the importance of all of these dimensions of a person's suffering and that good pain relief is unlikely without attention to all of these areas.

Patients with chronic or advanced disease face many losses—loss of normality, loss of health, and potential loss of the future. Physical symptoms impose limitations on lifestyle. In addition, the symptom can be interpreted as an ever-present reminder of the underlying disease. *Never* underestimate the power of feelings in a patient's suffering and always seek to understand the *impact* of the symptom. This will help you set some goals with the patient that are meaningful in improving the quality of their life.

> **Rule 3: Always consider the multidimensional (holistic) context of patients' symptoms.**

Deciding what treatment to use is based on evidence—evidence of the mechanism of the symptom and evidence of the treatment's efficacy and safety in that situation. Later in this chapter we give you some of the evidence. For example:

- 5-HT$_3$ antagonists are highly effective in the treatment of nausea of chemotherapy because of their effect on the chemoreceptor trigger zone and the gut. They are less effective than metoclopramide as an antiemetic for the nausea of gastric stasis.

- A distressing cough in a Motor Neurone Disease (MND) patient with aspiration pneumonia may be helped by antibiotics to reduce the generation of phlegm, physiotherapy to aid expectoration, and antitussive measures that include opioids that act on the brain stem cough reflex (e.g. methadone and pholcodeine). Oropharyngeal local anaesthetic (spray or nebulized) may be helpful for patients in the last days of life to reduce the triggering of the cough reflex.

- A patient who is fearful of dying may be helped more by discussing and addressing specific fears rather than taking benzodiazepines.

> **Rule 4: Use treatments that address the mechanism of the symptom**

Explanation and information

Research and common sense tell us that most people wish to know what is going on with their bodies: what is happening and what to expect. This usually reduces the patient's anxieties, even if it confirms their worst suspicions. (A monster in the light is usually better faced than a monster unseen in the shadows.) A clear, sensitive explanation and discussion of the suggested treatments and follow-up plan is important for the patient to gain a sense of control and security and help them to share in decision making. Your skills in communication will be needed here (see Chapter 2).

> **Rule 5: Management of a problem should always begin with sensitive explanation and discussion of the findings and what this means**

Individualized treatment

The individual physical, social, and psychological circumstances of the patient and their views and wishes should be considered in planning care. This is why you need to share treatment options with patients. Don't come to them with a predetermined plan that they should comply with. When you get good at this, you can even ask them first what they have in mind, what will make the biggest difference to them, what's most important.

> **Rule 6: Treatments work best if they suit the individual patient**

For example:

♦ The compression bandages for Mrs Stevens' lymphoedema treatment may be unused unless there is someone available to help her fit them daily.

♦ Mrs Jones may decline admission to get on top of her pain unless someone looks after her cat.

♦ Mr Singh may decline opioids because he wishes his mind to be clear on his journey towards death and the next life.

♦ Dr Peters had severe nausea with chemotherapy, pregnancy, and buprenorphine in the past. Starting an opioid for her pain control will need to take this into account and will require use of a prophylactic antiemetic.

Re-evaluation and supervision

Symptoms can change frequently in advanced disease, especially when patients are frail. New problems can occur and established ones worsen. Proactive follow-up is vital.

If you have prescribed something to improve symptoms, check on its beneficial and adverse effects the next day. Getting on top of symptoms usually requires a few days of review and adjustment of medications or other measures. Sometimes more information from investigations is required. If things are not improving, asking a specialist palliative care team for additional advice is important. There should be specialist teams in the community and hospital settings. Often they are linked to hospices (see Chapter 8).

> **Rule 7: Check to see that what you have done has worked**

 LEARNING EXERCISE

How does the hospital or primary care team you are working in now seek specialist palliative care advice? Ask your senior colleagues and look for information leaflets in your area.

Rule 8: Seek specialist advice if problems are not improving

Both the patient and health care team should know exactly who the patient or carer will contact if problems arise in future, especially out of normal working hours. Will there be a regular system for review? It is often useful to discuss with the patient and carer under what circumstances, and where, the patient should be admitted. Plans need to be communicated clearly with all those involved if the patient's wishes are to drive care decisions.

Rule 9: Plan follow-up and the safety net

Attention to detail

The quality of palliative care is in the detail of care. For instance, it is vital to ensure that the patient not only has a prescription for the correct drug but also that he or she can obtain it from the pharmacy, has adequate supplies to cover a weekend, and understands how to adjust it if the problem worsens. Symptom control can be so finely balanced that the smallest of errors can make all the difference to the outcome.

Attention to detail is important in all of the aspects of symptom control previously outlined. Without it, resources and effort may be wasted and patients may continue to suffer needlessly.

Continuing to care and providing continuity

It can be difficult for professionals to continue to make the time to care for patients in the very last stage of their lives. How do you prioritize this when patients who are acutely ill need the attention? Often, however, these patients are avoided because it is awkward and sad and we feel that there is nothing we can do.

> During ward rounds the four 'caring' consultants conducted comprehensive consultations and showed a holistic approach to care. Attention was paid to both the physical and psychosocial needs of patients . . . The remaining 10 consultants concentrated on the patient's disease, the physical deterioration . . . there was minimal or no personal contact with the patients . . . When active medical intervention was scaled down and death was imminent they withdrew from the patient, either remaining at the foot of the bed or passing the patient's bed without comment or with a brief aside . . . 'no change?' or 'still there?'[2]

> Reproduced from Mills, M. et al., Care of dying patients in hospital, *British Medical Journal*, Volume 309, Number 6954, pp. 583–6, Copyright © 1994, with permission from BMJ Publishing Group.

Helplessness is an uncomfortable feeling. We like to be able to 'do' things. However, it is important to remember the great value to the patient and their carers in continuing to stay involved, to acknowledge how difficult the situation is, and not to abandon the patient because it is painful and distressing for the professional.

> **Rule 10: Patients who are dying, and their families, need professionals to demonstrate that they continue to care for them as people, and that this care is an important part of their job**

Continuity of care is also vital. No professional can be available 24/7 but transfer of important information about the patient, to doctors and others who take over the responsibility of care, is vital. Some ways of doing this are:

- speaking to the doctor on call;
- sending information to out-of-hours services (with the patient's permission);
- clear notes to inform any health care professional;
- a summary letter held by the patient;
- patient-held records;
- providing contact details for the key health care team (see Rule 9).

The management of pain

The successful management of pain can be one of the most satisfying experiences for a healthcare professional. The *good news* is that in over 80% of patients with cancer-related pain, it can be well controlled using low-cost, low-technology, straightforward methods. This probably holds true for most patients with pain related to non-malignant conditions. The *bad news* is that, in general, this is not achieved for patients. Key factors in this are the knowledge, skills, and attitudes of professionals.

Remember that pain is always a physical and emotional experience. Lots of factors influence pain and how a patient copes with it, and the concept of total pain is covered in Chapter 3. The management of cancer-related pain is outlined in Figure 5.3.

 THINK POINT

Studies in the United Kingdom, United States, and Europe have shown that almost 50% of people with cancer-related pain receive inadequate relief.

World Health Organization (WHO) analgesic ladder

Although the WHO analgesic ladder (Figure 5.2)[3] was developed for use in cancer pain, a stepwise approach, using a limited number of drugs, is probably equally applicable to the management of chronic pain in advanced disease due to other causes, and has the potential to simplify prescribing. However, the use of strong opioids in non-malignant chronic pain is a controversial area and requires specialist advice and supervision.

The WHO approach *combines* two modalities of pain relief—non-opioids and opioids.

◆ Non-opioid analgesics such as non-steroidal anti-inflammatory drugs (NSAIDs) or paracetamol reduce inflammation and/or prostaglandin synthesis and, thereby, reduce stimulation of nociceptors on peripheral nerves.

◆ Opioids reduce transmission of nociceptive stimuli to the conscious brain through inhibition at opioid receptors in the brain stem, spinal cord, and, perhaps, in peripheral nerves.

WHO Analgesic ladder

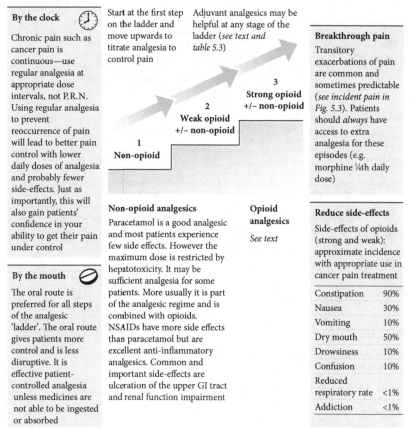

By the clock

Chronic pain such as cancer pain is continuous—use regular analgesia at appropriate dose intervals, not P.R.N. Using regular analgesia to prevent reoccurrence of pain will lead to better pain control with lower daily doses of analgesia and probably fewer side-effects. Just as importantly, this will also gain patients' confidence in your ability to get their pain under control

By the mouth

The oral route is preferred for all steps of the analgesic 'ladder'. The oral route gives patients more control and is less disruptive. It is effective patient-controlled analgesia unless medicines are not able to be ingested or absorbed

Start at the first step on the ladder and move upwards to titrate analgesia to control pain

Adjuvant analgesics may be helpful at any stage of the ladder (*see text and table 5.3*)

1 Non-opioid

2 Weak opioid +/– non-opioid

3 Strong opioid +/– non-opioid

Non-opioid analgesics

Paracetamol is a good analgesic and most patients experience few side effects. However the maximum dose is restricted by hepatotoxicity. It may be sufficient analgesia for some patients. More usually it is part of the analgesic regime and is combined with opioids. NSAIDs have more side effects than paracetamol but are excellent anti-inflammatory analgesics. Common and important side-effects are ulceration of the upper GI tract and renal function impairment

Opioid analgesics

See text

Breakthrough pain

Transitory exacerbations of pain are common and sometimes predictable (*see incident pain in Fig. 5.3*). Patients should *always* have access to extra analgesia for these episodes (e.g. morphine ¹⁄₆th daily dose)

Reduce side-effects

Side-effects of opioids (strong and weak): approximate incidence with appropriate use in cancer pain treatment

Constipation	90%
Nausea	30%
Vomiting	10%
Dry mouth	50%
Drowsiness	10%
Confusion	10%
Reduced respiratory rate	<1%
Addiction	<1%

Figure 5.2 The WHO analgesic ladder for cancer pain management[3]

Adapted with permission from WHO's *Cancer Pain Ladder for Adults*, Copyright © World Health Organization, available from <http://www.who.int/cancer/palliative/painladder/en/>.

Think—what is the cause of each of this patient's pains?	For each pain note: • characteristics • site • radiation • severity • onset • exacerbating and relieving factors • effects of any drugs tried • impact on the patient	What investigations may help? E.g. X-ray, bone scan
In the light of your assessment, what are the best drug and non-drug strategies for pain control?	Non-drug approaches include: • TENS • relaxation • hypnosis • acupuncture • radiotherapy • surgery Pattern recognition (*see table below*)	The WHO analgesic ladder (see Fig. 5.3)
Use a multi-professional, holistic, team approach	Ask the patient or nurse to use a pain chart to assess progress	Physio- and occupational therapists are essential for managing incident pain	Plan when and who will make sure there is satisfactory progress
Explain to patient and family and review the patient early	What does this pain mean to the patient?	Many people feel that severe pain is inevitable in cancer, and this may lead to fear, suffering, and reluctance to ask for help. Pain may be erroneously interpreted by patients as an indication of progression of their cancer and therefore a signal of their approaching death

Recognize patterns of pain

Type of pain	Key features	Response to opioids	Comments
Soft tissue	Localized ache throbbing, gnawing	Good	>80% pain control easily achievable by non-opioid ± opioid
Visceral	Poorly localized deep ache. Pain may be referred to specific sites	Good	>80% pain control easily achievable by non-opioid ± opioid
Bone	Well localized aching pain, local tenderness	Variable	Non-steroid anti-inflammatory drugs (NSAIDs) + radiotherapy are important treatment options
Neuropathic (*see text*)	Difficult to describe; dysaesthesia; associated motor/sensory loss; pain distributed in specific dermatomal, radicular, or nerve territory	Often poor	Adjuvant treatments usually needed; early referral for specialist advice improves outcome
Incident pain	Occurs episodically: on movement, weight bearing, change of dressing, etc.	Moderate	Find ways to avoid provocation. Consider: • extra analgesics before predictable provocation • gaseous nitrous oxide • spinal routes of analgesia • orthopaedic interventions for spinal stabilization and strengthening weight-bearing bones

> **If you need any help with a patient you can contact the palliative care team in hospital or community**

Figure 5.3 A guide to the successful management of cancer-related pain

However, as indicate in the table 'Recognize patterns of pain' in Figure 5.3, a variable response to opioids should be anticipated and, in some patients, the addition of adjuvant analgesic agents is important in achieving pain control.

Weak opioid analgesics

Codeine and dihydrocodeine are used in combination with a non-opioid analgesic, such as paracetamol, at the second step of the ladder. Tablets containing a combination of weak opioids and paracetamol are readily available. There is a 'ceiling' to the effect of weak opioids (usually two tablets, four times daily) and if regular, maximum doses do not achieve adequate analgesia, then you should take a step up the ladder, i.e. the weak opioid should be replaced with a strong opioid, usually morphine.

Tramadol and tapentadol may have a place on this step of the ladder for some patients.

Strong opioid analgesics

In the United Kingdom, morphine, derived from opium, is the strong opioid of first choice. When using morphine and other strong opioids, the following points should be remembered:

- Explain the drug to the patient and their carer. Anticipate that they may have significant concerns, which need to be addressed.[4]
- Prevention of side-effects: use a prophylactic stimulant laxative such as senna or macrogol; consider an antiemetic.

 LEARNING EXERCISE

What worries people about using morphine?

- Write a list of ten things you anticipate that your patients may be worried about when you suggest they start morphine.
- Now think how you will alleviate their worries.
- Check these thoughts out with the next patient you see who is on, or about to start, morphine for chronic pain.
- What might worry *you*? How might you put patients at risk and how will you ensure good risk management? There are risks both in prescribing too little and too much morphine. Read on to reduce your worries about this and increase your competence.

Using morphine: Step 1, gain control of pain

◆ Titrate the dose needed for pain relief by using either oral sustained-release morphine, 12 hourly, or oral immediate-release morphine (elixir or tablets), 4 hourly. A total daily dose of 20–30 mg is the starting dose recommended by NICE[4]. This may need to be higher for those patients that have been on maximal dose weaker opioids. In the elderly or those with renal impairment, smaller doses (2.5 mg, 4 hourly) and closer monitoring are required.

◆ Ensure that patients have access to immediate-release morphine for break-through pain on an as-required (PRN) basis. The dose is 1/6th of the total daily dose of morphine.

◆ Reassess pain control daily.

◆ Titrate the dose to achieve pain relief by a 30–50% increment in dose, or to incorporate the PRN doses that the patient has needed to use.

◆ Remember to increase the PRN dose for breakthrough pain as you increase the regular dose by calculating 1/6th of new total daily dose.

◆ A 'diary' of treatment and its effect is helpful in titration if the patient is at home.

◆ If your patient's pain does not improve within 3 days, or there are severe side-effects, seek specialist help.

> ### ? THINK POINT
>
> ◆ Two-thirds of patients with cancer pain need less than 200 mg morphine per day.
>
> ◆ One-third of patients may need higher doses, occasionally 1200 mg or more of morphine per day.

Using morphine: Step 2, maintenance of pain control

Most patients prefer to be on 12 hourly sustained-release preparations to mini-mize the medication burden.

If the patient's pain has improved *but* they have persistent morphine-related side-effects, these may be lessened by switching to an alternative strong opioid (you may want to seek specialist advice for this).

All patients on long-acting opioid preparations require an immediate-release, short-acting opioid to be available for episodes of breakthrough pain. This is usually morphine and the dose should be equivalent to 1/6th of the total daily dose (TDD).

Table 5.2 Conversion between oral morphine and subcutaneous (SC) diamorphine (3mg oral morphine = 1 mg SC diamorphine) and subcutaneous morphine (2 mg oral morphine = 1 mg SC morphine).

Opioid and route	Equivalent dose		
Oral morphine (mg/24 h)	90	180	240
SC diamorphine for infusion (mg/24 h)	30	60	80
SC diamorphine for breakthrough pain (mg) (1/6 TDD)	5	10	15
SC morphine for infusion (mg/24 h)	45	90	120
SC morphine for breakthrough pain (mg) (1/6 TDD)	7.5	15	20

Converting between strong opioids

This may be useful for patients who:

♦ require non-oral opioids (transdermal or subcutaneous infusion);

♦ have intolerable opioid-related side-effects, which may be drug specific;

♦ use high doses of opioids with apparent tolerance to its analgesic effects.

Except for conversion to subcutaneous morphine or diamorphine (shown in Table 5.2), this will usually require specialist advice.

Neuropathic pain and the use of adjuvant analgesics

Pain that arises because of damage to the nervous system is particularly unpleasant, often difficult for patients to describe, and problematic to manage. Specialist advice is frequently required and you should seek this early for any patient you think has neuropathic pain, since it seems that the longer it is left untreated, the harder it is to resolve.

Patients experience a variety of abnormal sensations in neuropathic pain, which have specific terminologies (Box 5.2). Differentiating these may give guidance to pathophysiology of the nerve damage and the best modality of treatment. Pain in an area of numbness or altered sensation is a pathognomonic indicator of neuropathic pain.

Nervous tissue may be damaged by a variety of insults, for example:

♦ infarction, e.g. central post-stroke pain;

♦ infection, e.g. HIV-related neuropathy;

♦ drugs, e.g. post-chemotherapy neuropathy;

♦ trauma, e.g. radiculopathy associated with spinal cord compression.

The management of such pains is largely an advanced subject, but you should be aware that the general approach is to employ the WHO analgesic ladder and that 'adjuvant' analgesics are frequently required.

Box 5.2 Abnormal sensations in neuropathic pain

Dysaesthesia: spontaneous and evoked abnormal sensation, e.g. pins and needles.

Hyperaesthesia: an increased (non-painful) sensitivity to non-painful stimulation, e.g. touch.

Hyperalgesia: increased response (intensity and duration) to a stimulus that is normally painful, e.g. pinch.

Allodynia: pain caused by a stimulus that is not normally painful, e.g. clothing in shingles.

Hyperpathia: explosive and often prolonged painful response to a non-painful stimulus.

An adjuvant analgesic is a drug that is not generally classified as an analgesic but has a pain-relieving effect in particular circumstances. The evidence base for the use of such drugs is often slim, and trials have been undertaken mostly in patients with trigeminal neuralgia, post-herpetic neuralgia, and diabetic neuropathy. Table 5.3 outlines the use of the key first-line adjuvant analgesic drugs. For many patients, unresolvable side-effects limit the dose of the drug, especially for patients who are also on opioids.

Table 5.3 Adjuvant analgesics for neuropathic pain

Drug group	Probable main mechanism of action	Typical regime
Tricyclic antidepressants	Enhance central inhibition by increase in synaptic serotonin	Amitriptyline 10–25 mg at night, increased slowly to a maximum of 75 mg/24 h Duloxetine 30–60 mg/day, increased up to maximum of 120 mg/24 h
Anticonvulsants	Decrease neuronal excitability	Carbamazepine 200 mg twice a day, increased slowly to a maximum of 1.2 g/24 h Gabapentin 100–300 mg at night, increased slowly to a maximum of 600 mg three times daily Pregabalin 50–75 mg twice daily, increased up to a maximum of 600 mg/24 h
Steroids	Reduce perineural oedema	Dexamethasone 6 mg in the morning Higher dose (16 mg) may be useful, e.g. in spinal cord compression

Nausea and vomiting

Like pain, the successful management of nausea is underpinned by first considering all the potential causes. Nausea and vomiting are often linked, but some patients may have one or the other. The characteristics or pattern of the patient's symptoms often gives an indication of the underlying cause. It may be possible to remove the cause, and the benefits and burdens of treatment should be weighed up with patients and the multidisciplinary team. For example, relieving intestinal obstruction through surgery might be technically possible but, in a very frail patient with disseminated metastases, it may cause deterioration which will lead to them dying post-surgery, in hospital. Treating a drowsy, nauseated patient who has hypercalcaemia with intravenous rehydration and bisphosphonate infusion, however, may restore a patient to a good quality of life for many months.

The management of nausea, based on suggested first-choice drugs for the various underlying causes, is outlined in Figure 5.4. Many patients will need the medication to be given by a non-oral route, at least initially. Non-drug treatments may, in addition, be useful for some patients. These include acupuncture, acupressure 'Sea' bands, relaxation, hypnosis, and reflexology.

For some patients, you may not be able to work out what the underlying cause is from your consideration of the characteristics and from investigations. In addition a few patients experience intractable nausea which dose not respond well enough to first and second line treatment. It is useful, for these patients, to think more deeply about the neurophysiology of nausea and vomiting. Figure 5.5 outlines an approach to prescribing in these situations.

Breathlessness and cough

Breathlessness in advanced malignant and non-malignant disease is frequently chronic and refractory. It persists at rest or on minimal activity despite optimal management of the underlying disease process. It has a profound impact on patients, disrupting their day-to-day functioning and causing social isolation.

The terms dyspnoea, breathlessness, and shortness of breath are often used interchangeably. Breathlessness is the term most often used by patients. Breathlessness is a symptom that can only be described and interpreted by the patient and, like pain, its intensity and impact is subjective. The degree of breathlessness that a patient experiences may not align with physiological parameters that you might measure (respiratory rate, oxygen saturations, and the use of accessory muscles) and is a complex interaction between a range of factors (Figure 5.6). Figure 5.7 gives an outline for the management of breathlessness and the related symptom cough in advanced disease.

Think—why is this patient vomiting?	Only by making a reasoned judgement as to the cause of a patient's vomiting do you stand a chance of controlling this common symptom. Consider:
	• the disease process itself
	• complications of the disease process
	• side-effects of drugs
	• previous drugs used
	• complications of other treatments
	• psychosocial factors
	• the characteristics of the nausea and vomiting

In the light of your assessment; reverse the reversible, use the most appropriate non-drug and drug methods to control it (see table)

Classifications	Causes*	Characteristics	First choice drugs	Alternative drugs
Upper GI stasis/outflow obstruction	• tumour • anticholinergic drugs • hepatomegaly	• epigastric discomfort • worse on eating • eased by vomiting • variable nausea	*metoclopramide 10–20 mg TDS oral 30–60 mg/24 h SC	domperidone 10–20 mg TDS oral 30–60 mg PR 12 h
Chemically induced	• drugs • metabolic • toxic	• constant nausea • variable vomiting	haloperidol 1.5–5 mg oral 1.5–5 mg/24 h SC	metoclopromide 10–20 mg t.d.s. oral 30–60 mg/24 h SC
Constipation	• drugs • because of cancer • immobility	• nausea and faeculant vomiting • associated with constipation	stimulant and softener laxative (eg Macrogol, 1 sachet in the morning)	laxative and glycerine or bisacodyl suppositories
Raised intracranial pressure	• cerebral mets • cerebral haemorrhage	• nausea worse in the morning • projectile vomiting • worse on head movement	trial of steroids Dexamethasone 8–16 mg/24 h oral/SC/IM/IV	Cyclizine 25–50 mg t.d.s. oral 100–150 mg/24 h
Intestinal obstruction	• malignant • non malignant	• vomiting with abdominal pain, distension and constipation	hyoscine butylbromide 60–200 mg/24 h SC	trial of octreotide 200 µg up to 600 µg/24 h SC
Anxiety	• any cause	• symptoms worse when anxious	Diazepam 2–5 mg t.d.s.	
Unknown cause	If you cannot discern a reason for your patient's nausea and vomiting		Cyclizine 25–50 mg t.d.s. oral 100–150 mg/24 h SC	

* **Remember: many causes can be treated without long-term anti-emetics** (e.g. stopping causative drugs, treating constipation, reversing metabolic disturbance, treating infection, surgical treatment, etc.)

t.d.s., three times daily; SC, subcutaneously; IM, intramuscularly; IV, intravenously; PR, per rectum or rectal

*metoclopramide can cause pakinsonian and other dystonic side effects and caution is needed in longer term and higher dose use. Maximum dose 500 mcg/kg

If prescribing an anti-emetic, then must have a very good reason to use oral route

Explain to patient and family and review the patient early

If you need any help with a patient you can contact the palliative care team in hospital or community

Figure 5.4 A guide to the management of nausea

Although the principles described in figure 5.4 will be successful in many cases there are some cases where control is harder to achieve. Then you may need to prescribe more than one anti-emetic, or use different drugs. When doing this it helps if you understand the neurophysiology, so that you don't prescribe inappropriately.

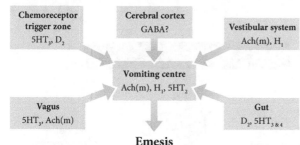

Receptor site affinities of selected anti-emetics							
Drug name	D_2	H_1	Ach(m)	$5HT_2$	$5HT_3$	$5HT_4$	GABA
Metoclopramide	• •	–	–	–	–	•	–
Domperidone	• •	–	–	–	–	–	–
Ondansetron	–	–	–	–	• • •	–	–
Cyclizine	–	• •	• •	–	–	–	–
Hyoscine	–	–	• • •	–	–	–	–
Haloperidol	• • •	–	–	–	–	–	–
Prochlorperazine	• •	•	•	•	–	–	–
Levomepromazine	• •	• •	• •	• • •	–	–	–
Diazepam	–	–	–	–	–	–	• •

Key

D_2	Dopamine type 2 receptors
H_1	Histamine type 1 receptors
Ach(m)	Muscarinic cholinergic
$5HT_{2,3,4}$	Serotonin type 2, 3 and 4
GABA	Gamma-amino-butyric acid
–	no affinity
•	slight affinity
• •	moderate affinity
• • •	marked affinity

Useful points:

- Don't use the IM route if you can help it—it's painful!
- Ensure any anti-emetic used is given regularly: anti-emetics as required are never going to control regular nausea and vomiting
- Use any anti-emetic to maximum dose (if side effects permit) before swapping
- If first drug is unsuccessful, try one from a different group
- If a second drug is unsuccessful combine two antiemetics from differing groups
- Don't use two drugs from the same group ot the same time
- Haloperidol and Cyclizine are often a successful combination
- Anti-cholinergic drugs have predictable side effects and can antagonise metochlopromide and other prokinetic drugs
- Consider non-drug methods (e.g. acupuncture, ginger, relaxation, hypnotherapy, control malodour, avoid certain foods, small meals)
- Pain and coughing can cause vomiting
- For intractable vomiting it may be worth trying:
  - Levomepromazine 6.25–25 mg OD orally or 6.25–12.5 mg/24 h SC
  - three day trial of dexamethasone 4–12 mg/24 h
  - three day trial of ondansetron 8 mg BD or TDS

> If you need any help with a patient you can contact the palliative care team in hospital or community

Figure 5.5 Management of intractable vomiting

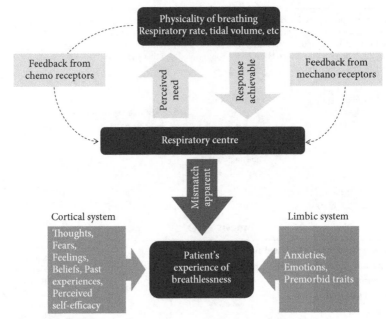

Figure 5.6 Mechanisms of breathlessness in advanced disease

Reproduced from Powell, B., Managing breathlessness in advanced disease, *Clinical Medicine,* Volume 14, Number 3, pp. 308–311, Copyright © 2014 by the Royal College of Physicians. Reproduced with permission.

Constipation and diarrhoea

Managing constipation generally isn't rocket science, although occasionally it can feel as if it needs that sort of propulsion to get them moving! The biggest issue is that health care professionals fail to give patients prophylactic laxatives (vital with opioids) and don't ask patients how their bowels are. It is important you know the potential side-effects on the bowel of any of the drugs prescribed for patients, warn the patients, and ensure laxatives are prescribed in advance of a problem developing.

Diarrhoea is a less common side-effect of drugs used in palliative care and in patients with advanced disease. It can be very troublesome for those that do have it and may lead to social restrictions, odour, mountains of washing, and very sore skin. Figure 5.8 outlines the management of these two problems.

Symptom management in the last days of life

Dying people require a truly holistic approach to their care. Many physical problems arise and comfort is essential, but so too is consideration of place of care,

Think—why is the patient short of breath?	There is often more than one cause for dyspnoea. **Common causes** to consider are:
	• Anxiety
	• Lung cancer (primary or secondary)
	    • Obstruction of bronchus
	    • Effusion
	• Anaemia
	• Concurrent lung disease
	• Loss of respiratory muscle
	• Splinting of diaphragm
	• Pulmonary embolus
	
	If possible watch the patient walk: it tells you a lot.
		When to order tests? This can be tricky. Chest X-ray, full blood count, and sputum microbiology may be useful diagnostically.

In the light of your assessment; reverse the reversible, use the most appropriate non-drug and drug methods to control it (see table) Listening, understanding and reassuring are vitally important	**Specific treatment for specific causes**	
	Anxiety	General measures and lorazepam (see below)
	Lung cancer	• Speak to oncologist about radiotherapy, chemotherapy • Consider pleural drainage if effusion present
	Anaemia	Consider transfusion. Always check; did they improve and for how long?
	Concurrent lung disease	Antibiotics (infection), Bronchodilators (COPD/asthma), diuretics (CCF), etc.
	Loss of respiratory muscle	General measures (see below)
	Splinting of diaphragm	Drain ascites if present, otherwise general measures and non-specific drug options (see below)
	Pulmonary embolus	Anticoagulation sometimes appropriate in very advanced disease. Analgesia and general measures

Non-specific treatment for general symptom control

General measures; can be considered in all patients whatever the cause	• Give the patient time and reassurance • Relaxation • Breathing techniques • Open window or fan • Positioning for maximal breathing • Consider physio or occupational therapy referral
Non-specific drug options	• Lorazepam 0.5 mg PRN sublingually. • Morphine 1–2.5 mg every 4 hours if not on opioids, titrating up according to response. If on opioids, make a 30–50% increase in dose. • Oxygen. In the hypoxic (PaO2 <9)

What about cough?
• Treat the cause; cancer, antibiotics, diuretics, bronchodilators
• Nebulized saline if tenacious sputum
• Simple linctus 5 ml, 3–4 times a day
• Codeine linctus 5–10 ml, 3–4 times a day

Involve the patient and key individuals in all stages and agree follow-up

COPD, chronic obstructive pulmonary disease; CCF, congestive cardiac failure.

If you need any help with a patient you can contact the palliative care team in hospital or community

Figure 5.7 The management of breathlessness and cough in advanced disease

Constipation

Remember this is a common problem so always ask about it. Common causes are:
• drugs, especially opioids
• poor oral intake
• immobility
• gut cancers
• co-morbidity
  (e.g. diverticular disease)

Think—why has this patient got constipation or diarrhoea?

Diarrhoea

Common causes to think about are:
• over use of laxatives
• other drugs (e.g. antibiotics)
• constipation with overflow
• side-effect of pelvic radiotherapy
• malabsorption from bowel resections or pancreatic malfunction
• tumour invasion of gut wall
• infection
• fistula
• co-morbidity

• reverse the cause if possible
• always prescribe a laxative with an opioid
• titrate the dose up to get a result
• think carefully and consider patient's embarrassment

Laxatives
• As a prophylactic measure consider senna tablets (1–3 daily). For established constipation use macrogol if patient can tolerate the volume of water required for administration (and the sodium load); or consider sodium picosulphate 5–30 ml/day or bisocodyl or sometimes co-danthrusate.

Rectal treatments
(may or may not be needed)
• *hard faeces*: soften with glycerine suppositories
• *soft faeces*: stimulate with bisacodyl suppositories
• *empty rectum*: consider obstruction or phosphate enema

In the light of your assessment, what are the best strategies for good symptom control?

Liaise closely with rest of team when making decision Involve the patient and their carers as much as possible in the decision making and be clear about follow-up

Cause	Treatment
laxatives, antibiotics, antacids, chemotherapy	stop drugs if possible
constipation with overflow	laxatives and suppositories/ enemas
malabsorption	pancreatic supplements, bilary stenting
tumour invasion of gut wall	palliative radiotherapy or chemotherapy
infection	treatment guided by culture and sensitivity
co-morbidity	treat according to condition
cause unknown or specific treatment ineffective	Loperamide up to 16 mg daily Codeine 10–60 mg daily Octreotide SC (seek specialist advice)

Remember:
Oral rehydration, low-fibre diet and the importance of good nursing care

---

If you need any help with a patient you can contact the palliative care team in hospital or community

Figure 5.8 The management of constipation and diarrhoea in advanced disease

their need for religious ritual or prayer, and support for their relatives. Attention to detail and continued involvement of the clinical team are paramount. The non-physical aspects of care have been discussed in other chapters. You should take the approach outlined in Figure 5.9 for the physical aspects of their care.

Drugs commonly used in palliative care

A wide range of drugs is available for symptom management. We suggest that you gain familiarity and a good working knowledge of a relatively small group that you may need on a frequent basis. You need to know when to use them, common and important side-effects, cautions and interactions, and methods of administration. You should use other textbooks to familiarize yourself with their pharmacology.

Analgesics

Step 1: Non-opioids

- Paracetamol
- Ibuprofen

Step 2: Opioids for mild to moderate pain

- Codeine

Step 3: Opioids for severe pain

- Morphine
- Diamorphine

Adjuvants

- Amitriptyline
- Pregabalin

Antiemetics

- Metoclopramide
- Haloperidol
- Cyclizine

Anticholinergics

- Glycopyrronium
- Hyoscine butylbromide

Is the patient dying?	Patients who are dying may often be:

- profoundly weak
- gaunt
- drowsy
- disorientated

- having difficulty taking things orally
- breathing in abnormal patterns

- unable to concentrate
- reducing peripheral perfusion with skin colour and temperature changes

---

Is he/she comfortable?

What do I need to decide?

What should I anticipate?

General considerations

Review drip, drugs, and other interventions
Can you stop:
- drugs
- IV fluids
- blood tests
- routine observations?

It is likely that many are not helpful at this stage.

Route of drug administration
- Use syringe driver for SC medications *(see Chapter 6)*.
- Use NSAID per rectum (PR) for stiffness and bone pain.

Common symptoms

PAIN:
see section management of pain and Figure 5.3
Nausea:
see section Nausea and vomiting and Figures 5.4 and 5. 5
Breathlessness:
see section breathlessness and cough and Figure 5.7

Extreme fatigue
Patients need anyone and everyone to help with a drink or repositioning a pillow

Excess respiratory secretions
- optimize the patient's position in bed
- very occasionally suction is helpful
- use an anticholinergic agent:
  Glycopyrronium 200mcg stat and 600–1200 mcg/24 h
  Hyoscine butylbromide SC 20 mg stat: 60–120 mg/24 h
  Hyoscine hydrobromide SC 200 µg stat: 600–1200 mg/24 h

Mouth care
- Hourly nursing attention
- Water based gel to lips
- Sips of water if possible moisten tongue with water

Terminal restlessness and agitation
The reasons may be multiple, E.g. hypotension, hypoxia, biochemical abnormalities.
Most patients are very frightened.
It is very distressing to carers.
It is perhaps the most difficult symptom to manage at home.
- Exclude an obvious cause for distress
  (e.g. full bladder, wet bed.)
- Reassure the patient and talk to the family about what is happening.
- Try and establish a quiet, low-stimulation environment for the patient.

Have I talked to the patient and the relatives?

See Chapters 2, 3 and 4

Medication, usually parenteral, may be needed if the patient is a danger to him/herself or clearly very distressed:

Where delirium and psychotic features are predominant:
haloperidol SC 5 mg stat and 5–10 mg/24 h
or
levomepromazine SC 12.5–25 mg stat or 12.5–100 mg/24 h

Where anguish and anxiety are predominant:
midazolam 2.5–5 mg stat then 5–30 mg/24 h
or
diazepam 5–10 mg PR

If you need any help with a patient you can contact the palliative care team in hospital or community

Figure 5.9 The management of physical symptoms in the last days of life

Steroids

- Dexamethasone
- Prednisolone

Sedatives

- Midazolam
- Haloperidol
- Levomepromazine

Laxatives

- Senna
- Macrogol

 SUMMARY BOX

- Pain, fatigue, breathlessness, and other symptoms are all very common in advanced disease of any nature. However, these are often undertreated and cause patients a lot of suffering.
- A holistic, multi professional approach will provide the best assessment and management of symptoms.
- The principles of symptom management are anticipation, assessment, explanation, individualized treatment, attention to detail, re-evaluation, and continuity of care.
- Good symptom management can be achieved, for most patients, by application of core knowledge and the effective use of a small group of drugs. Some patients have more complex problems and, in these cases, you will need the assistance of the specialist palliative care team.

Case history exercise: some thoughts on the issues to anticipate and forward plan for Petunia

The common issues that might arise for Petunia are:

- Pain: may need NSAIDs, opioids, and radiotherapy.
- Spinal cord compression: needs a neurological examination if she says she is unsteady or 'numb' or has a band of pain around the trunk.

- Anxiety about her young children: may need help, both practically and in telling the children.
- Work: may need advice regarding finances, benefits, and employment.
- Hypercalcaemia: check blood if nauseated or confused.

It is important that you are competent in assessing, diagnosing, and managing potential spinal cord compression. If you suspect spinal cord compression, then you must seek urgent oncological assessment. For further information, refer to the *Handbook of Palliative Care* (see 'Further reading' for details).

 KEY POINTS

To provide good symptom control you will have to:

- **Think**: what is causing this?
- **Understand**: how does it cause that?
- **Know**: what are the best treatment(s) for this cause?
- **Weigh up**: the benefits and burdens of treatment for this patient
- **Discuss**: sharing your findings and thoughts with the patient is an important therapeutic step. It helps them have more control to make decisions with you about the best approach for them.

You need to have familiarity with the prescribing and use of a small group of drugs, including controlled drugs.

You may need to ask for help from the specialist palliative care team if symptoms don't improve within a few days or for more complex problems.

References

1. **Abraham, A.** (2011) *Care and Compassion? Ten Investigations into Care of Older People.* Parliamentary and Health Service Ombudsman. London, The Stationery Office.
2. **Mills, M., Davies, H.T.O. and Macrae, W.A.** (1994) Care of dying patients in hospital. *British Medical Journal*; **309**:583–6.
3. **World Health Organization** (1996). *Cancer Pain Relief.* Geneva, WHO.
4. NICE (2012) *NICE Clinical Guideline 140*. Opioids in palliative care: safe and effective prescribing of strong opioids for pain in palliative care of adults. Manchester, National Institute for Health and Clinical Excellence.

Further reading

Faull, C., De Ceastecker, S., Nicholson, A., and Black, F. (eds) (2012) *Handbook of Palliative Care* (3rd edn). New Jersey, Wiley-Blackwell.

Palliative Care Adult Network Guidelines. Available at <http://book.pallcare.info/index.php>

The British Pain Society. (2010) *Cancer Pain Management. A Perspective from the British Pain Society, Supported by the Association for Palliative Medicine and the Royal College of General Practitioners.* London, The British Pain Society. Available from: <www.britishpainsociety.org> (accessed 6 Mar 2011).

Twycross, R. and Wilcock, A. (2013) *Palliative Care Formulary.* Abingdon, Radcliffe Medical Press.

The syringe driver: a useful way to deliver drugs

The syringe driver: a useful way to deliver drugs

The administration of drugs by subcutaneous infusion

It is quite common that patients with advanced illness cannot take their medications orally. This is always a good time for us to review the necessity to continue all drugs, many of which can be stopped at this time. However, maintaining good symptom management may require established medications (such as analgesics) to continue, or the addition of other medicines. An alternative to the oral route of drug delivery is needed to ensure effective symptom management is maintained. Some drugs can be given rectally (PR) but many require, or the patient would prefer, parenteral administration. The subcutaneous (SC) route is less painful than intramuscular (IM) and much more convenient than intravenous (IV).

In palliative care in the United Kingdom, using a small, battery-operated, portable infusion pump, usually referred to as a 'syringe driver', has become a firmly established method of administering a continuous subcutaneous infusion (CSCI) of analgesic, antiemetic, sedative, or anticholinergic drugs. For some patients, this is an interim measure while problems such as vomiting are controlled; for others, it is a way of delivering medicines to ensure comfort in the last days of their life.

This chapter will discuss the practicalities both of the use of the syringe driver and of the administration of drugs by subcutaneous infusion, and will help you to work through the following 'case history exercise'.

 CASE HISTORY EXERCISE

Jane has advanced cancer of the lung. She has been admitted to the ward today with nausea and vomiting, which she has been suffering from for the last 2 days. She is very frail. She has been taking sustained-release morphine, 40 mg 12 hourly, and because she hasn't kept this down, she is now in considerable pain. Her husband tells you that they know no further treatment will be possible and that they would, most of all, like to be at home, if only she can be more comfortable.

How can you manage Jane's symptoms to provide her with the best care?

Use of the syringe driver

The syringe driver delivers a continuous infusion of medication over a set period of time, usually 24 hours. There have been safety concerns relating to some syringe drivers that have their rate settings in millimetres (mm). As a result, the National Patient Safety Agency (NPSA) issued guidance to use syringe drivers with rate settings in ml per hour, with additional safety features.[1] These should be in place by December 2015. An example of a type of syringe driver with rate settings in ml/hr and safety features, commonly used in the United Kingdom, is the 'T34™ Ambulatory Syringe Pump' (see Figure 6.1). Medicines are drawn up into the syringe which is then attached to the pump, which is set to move the plunger of the syringe forward at an accurately controlled rate.

Syringe drivers allow patients to be as mobile as possible and avoid the necessity for repeated injections (important in frail, cachectic patients). They can be used in the hospital and at home and carried by the patient anywhere in their normal daily life.

The syringe driver delivers a continuous subcutaneous infusion (CSCI) which provides a steady plasma concentration of medicines. In this way, the

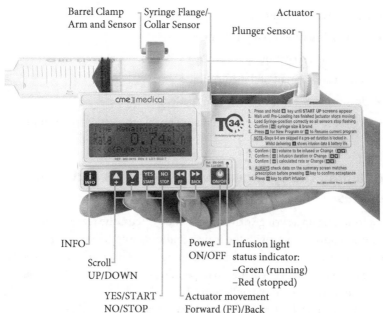

Figure 6.1 T34™ ambulatory syringe pump
Reproduced with permission of CME Medical, Copyright © 2014.

peaks and troughs of other delivery methods are avoided (see Box 6.1). Box 6.2 outlines some of the situations when a syringe driver should be considered.

Box 6.1 The advantages of using a syringe driver in comparison to intermittent injections

- Constant drug concentration
- Usually reloaded once in 24 hours
- No repeated injections
- Does not limit mobility
- Permits better control of nausea and vomiting
- Control of several symptoms with a combination of drugs in a single infusion

---

Box 6.2 Indications for using the syringe driver

- Persistent nausea and/or vomiting
- Difficulty in swallowing
- Mouth/throat/oesophageal lesions
- Intestinal obstruction
- Poor absorption of oral medication
- Unconscious and semi-conscious patients
- Profound weakness when patients are unable to swallow medication

---

Explaining the syringe driver to patients and their families

Prior to setting up a syringe driver, you should discuss the reasons for using the device and how it works with the patient and/or family. Some patients may find the syringe driver obtrusive and disconcerting. Some may have reservations and fear that a syringe driver equates to impending death. This may be because it is frequently used to deliver medications in the last days of life and, as such, is sometimes seen by both patients and staff as synonymous with a last rite. Some may even think that it hastens or causes death. This is a mistake. You may need to help them understand that the changes that are occurring in the patient

Box 6.3 Patient and family discussions

- Any past experience or knowledge about syringe drivers
- The stage of the illness and the reason for use of the syringe driver
- Any fears or anxieties about the syringe driver or the drugs to be used
- Explanation that the syringe driver allows symptoms to be managed but does not speed up the dying process
- Advance care planning
- Care of the syringe driver
- What to do and who to ask for help if the syringe driver is not working properly or if symptoms are not controlled
- The possible need to have extra (breakthrough) doses of medication, in addition to the syringe driver, to control symptoms

indicate an advanced stage of the patient's illness and the need for a syringe driver to help control their symptoms due to difficulty in taking oral medication.

In addition, some patients, earlier in their illness, may require a syringe driver to control symptoms for a short time and later convert back to oral medications. Whatever the reason, since staff, patients, and families may make wrongful assumptions about the use of syringe drivers, it is always important to explain the rationale for their use and the overall aims of care, invite questions, acknowledge anxieties, and reassure, where appropriate. Information leaflets may be useful but remember these should not replace discussion and personal explanation. The importance of open, honest discussion cannot be overstated. Topics you might want to include in discussions are included in Box 6.3.

Site of the infusion

Plastic cannulae (see Figure 6.2) are recommended, although metal butterfly needles can be used. The exact site where the needle will be placed under the skin should be influenced by the patient's preference and condition. Acceptable subcutaneous cannula insertion sites for use of the syringe driver are (see Figure 6.3):

- Anterior aspect of the upper arms or anterior abdominal wall
- Anterior aspect of the thigh
- The scapular, if the patient is distressed and/or agitated
- Anterior chest wall

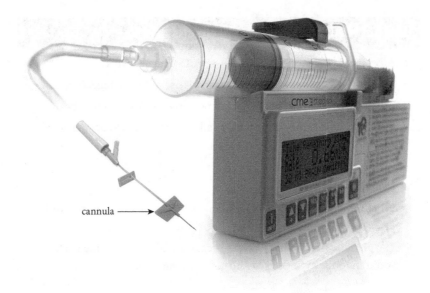

cannula

Figure 6.2 T34™ ambulatory syringe pump with cannula
Reproduced with permission of CME Medical, Copyright © 2014.

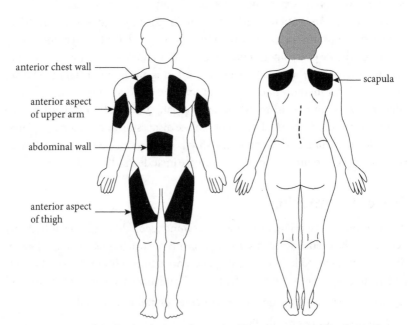

anterior chest wall

scapula

anterior aspect
of upper arm

abdominal wall

anterior aspect
of thigh

Figure 6.3 Areas of the body which are best suited for placement of the 'butterfly' needle or cannula to deliver the infusion
Adapted from Mark I. Johnson, *Transcutaneous Electrical Nerve Stimulation (TENS)*, Oxford University Press, Oxford, UK, Copyright © 2014, by permission of Oxford University Press.

Some places on the body are not suitable for insertion for reasons of poor absorption, discomfort, or increased risk of displacement. These are:

- Skin folds and breast tissue
- Directly over a tumour site
- Limbs with lymphoedema or oedema
- The abdominal wall, if ascites present
- Bony prominences
- Near a joint
- Infected, bruised, or broken skin
- An area which has previously been treated with radiotherapy

Starting the infusion

In most cases, a registered nurse who has received training in the use of the syringe driver will commence the subcutaneous infusion. It is not the place of this book to give guidance on how to do this. It is suggested that you refer to local policies and guidelines.

 LEARNING EXERCISE

Ask the nursing staff on your ward if you can watch them set up the next syringe driver.

Monitoring the infusion

Regular checks are required to be sure that the medication is being delivered correctly, preferably in conjunction with a dedicated syringe driver monitoring chart. Checks should include:

- Drugs and the doses
- Signs of redness, pain, or leakage at the site of the needle/cannula
- The rate is set correctly and the corresponding amount of fluid is infused
- Signs of precipitation of drugs (cloudiness) or crystallization
- Evidence of leakage from connections on the infusion and pump
- Ensure the tubing is not kinked
- The driver is working and the indicator light is flashing

Infusion site irritation

Site reactions are more likely to occur if the site is older than 72 hours or where the infusion contains cyclizine, levomopromazine, or high doses of diamorphine.[2] Should there be persistent problems with irritation at the injection site, consider:

◆ changing the site every 2–3 days, before reactions occur;

◆ reducing the concentration of drugs (i.e. larger volume);

◆ changing the drug or using an alternative route (some drugs are much more irritant than others);

◆ mixing drugs with 0.9% saline (if compatible);

◆ using a non-metal cannula;

◆ applying hydrocortisone 1% cream to the site around the needle and covering with an occlusive dressing.[3]

For more detailed discussion relating to site reactions and care of the syringe driver, a useful resource is Dickman and Schneider,[2] which provides a comprehensive guide.

Frequently asked questions

How long does it take for the infusion to begin working?

At least 4 hours. So, if the patient needs immediate interventions (e.g. for pain), they will require a stat (bolus) dose of relevant drugs given at the same time as commencing the subcutaneous continuous infusion.

How often should the infusion site be changed?

The infusion site should be changed when it is painful, appears inflamed or swollen. This will vary between patients and according to drug combinations being used. However, the site should be checked regularly, according to local policies, for signs of pain, inflammation, or swelling.[4]

What drugs can you deliver subcutaneously?

Although subcutaneous administration of the drugs indicated in Table 6.1 is common and accepted good practice in palliative care, the use of this route lies outside the product licence for most of these preparations. Only levomepromazine is licensed for subcutaneous use. This does not preclude their use in this way, but this is a particular clinical governance issue (see Chapter 7).

What drugs can you mix in the same syringe?

The main factor which affects compatibility of two or more drugs is their concentration, the pH of the solution, storage conditions, temperature, and strength.

Table 6.1 Drugs commonly used in a syringe driver for symptom management

Medication	Indication	SC starting dose per 24 hours
Analgesic		1/2 total daily dose of oral
Morphine		morphine
	Pain	10–20 mg (starting dose if not already taking opioids)
Diamorphine		1/3 total daily dose of oral morphine
		5–15 mg (starting dose if not already taking opioids)
		Increase dose, as needed, by 30% increments
Antiemetic		
Metoclopramide	Impaired gastric emptying Opioid-induced nausea	30 mg
Haloperidol	Drug-induced or metabolic cause of nausea	2.5–5 mg
Cyclizine	Intestinal obstruction	100–150 mg
Levomepromazine	Nausea	6.25–12.5 mg
Sedative		
Haloperidol	Terminal restlessness and agitation/delirium	2.5–5 mg
Midazolam	Terminal restlessness Myoclonic jerking Anticonvulsant	5–10 mg (up to 30 mg)
Levomepromazine	Terminal agitation and delirium	12.5–25 mg (up to 50 mg)
Anticholinergic		
Glycopyrronium	Terminal bronchial secretions	0.6 mg
Hyoscine hydrobromide (also antiemetic)		0.6 mg
Hyoscine butylbromide	Colic Intestinal obstruction	60 mg

Adapted with permission from Faull, C. et al., (Eds.), *Handbook of Palliative Care*, Third Edition, Wiley-Blackwell, Oxford, UK, Copyright © 2012, John Wiley and Sons.

Table 6.2 indicates the compatibility of two drug combinations used in palliative care. Where it is indicated that caution is required at higher concentrations, specialist pharmaceutical advice should be sought. In general, the combination of more than two drugs should be avoided without specialist advice.

What should be used to dilute the drugs?

In the United Kingdom, drugs are usually diluted with water for injections, unless there is a specific requirement to use 0.9% saline.[4]

Table 6.2 The compatibility of drugs combined in a syringe for SC infusion, using water for injection as diluent

	Morphine	Diamorphine	Metoclopramide	Haloperidol	Cyclizine	Levomepromazine	Midazolam	Glycopyrronium
Morphine		X	YES	YES (C)	YES	YES	YES	YES
Diamorphine	X		YES (C)	YES (C)	YES (C)	YES	YES	YES
Metoclopramide	YES	YES (C)		X	NO	X	YES	YES
Haloperidol	YES (C)	YES (C)	X		YES	X	YES	YES
Cyclizine	YES	YES (C)	NO	YES		YES	YES (C)	YES
Levomepromazine	YES	YES	X	X	YES		YES	YES
Midazolam	YES	YES	YES	YES	YES (C)	YES		YES
Glycopyronnium	YES	YES	YES	YES	YES	YES	YES	

C = caution at higher concentrations

X = generally not a clinically useful combination (same group of drug or counteracting effects)

Adapted with permission from Faull, C. et al., (Eds.), *Handbook of Palliative Care*, Third Edition, Wiley-Blackwell, Oxford, UK, Copyright © 2012, John Wiley and Sons.

Does the patient still need PRN doses?

Doses of medicine must always be prescribed for the patient to have should their symptoms, especially pain, be a problem.

What should I do if the dose of a drug needs to be changed?

Reviewing the patient's symptoms daily will often lead you to make changes to the prescription of drugs to achieve improvement in symptom management. If drug dosages need to be altered, the syringe should be recharged with the new prescription.

Case history exercise: some thoughts on the plan of management for Jane

In addition to your communication, assessment, and empathy skills, you will need to have the following knowledge and skills to manage Jane effectively:

- Safe use of the syringe driver for SC infusion.
- Calculation of the correct dose of SC morphine. For Jane, replacement of her sustained-release oral morphine requires 40 mg of SC morphine over 24 hours (i.e. 80mg ÷ 2). Because she is in pain, she will require a stat SC dose (1/6th total daily dose = 7.5 mg).
- Use of antiemetics by SC infusion. Consider haloperidol 2.5 mg/24 hours.
- Effective identification of possible causes for symptoms (e.g. hypercalcaemia) and whether reversal is possible However, you would need to discuss with the team if it would be appropriate to initiate treatment as this might be a terminal event which treatment will not alter.
- Effective prescribing of the multiple drugs that may be required to manage her symptoms.
- Effective identification of other needs (physical, psychological, social, financial, spiritual, practical, etc.).
- How to access specialist advice, support, and interventions for you and for Jane and her family.
- How to facilitate discussion with Jane and her husband about the future and to answer their questions and address their concerns.
- Optimal discharge planning, including district nurses to access a syringe driver in the community and change the infusion daily.
- Liaison with Jane's GP about the current situation and appropriate planning for future potential problems (e.g. referral to community palliative care team/hospice to avoid unwanted hospital admissions).

SUMMARY BOX

The syringe driver plays an important role in maintaining good symptom control when patients are no longer able to take oral medications. Patients and carers may have concerns about the syringe driver which we will need to discuss with them. Your knowledge of the benefits, use, and possible complications of the syringe driver will be important in helping you provide good care.

 KEY POINTS

To provide care for patients, with a syringe driver, you will need to know:

- when a syringe driver might be used to manage symptoms;
- what concerns the patients and carers may have, using your communications skills to help explore these and support them;
- how to use the syringe driver and monitor it;
- which drugs are commonly used in a syringe driver.

References

1. **National Patient Safety Agency.** (2010) Safer ambulatory syringe drivers. Available at: <http://www.nrls.npsa.nhs.uk/EasySiteWeb/getresource.axd?AssetID=92961&type=full&servicetype> (accessed on 3 Feb 2014).
2. **Dickman, A. and Schneider, J.** (2011) *The Syringe Driver: Continuous Subcutaneous Infusions in Palliative Care* (3rd edn). Oxford, Oxford University Press.
3. **Twycross, R. and Wilcock, A.** (2011) *Palliative Care Formulary* (4th edn). Oxford, Oxford Medical Press.
4. **Hirsch, C. and McKenna, M.** (2012) The syringe driver and medicines management in palliative care. **In** Faull, C., de Caestecker, D., Nicholson, A., and Black, F. (eds). *Handbook of Palliative Care* (3rd edn). New Jersey, Wiley-Blackwell.

Further reading and resources

Watson, M., Lucas, C., Hoy, A., et al. (2011) *Palliative Care Guidelines Plus*. Available at: <http://book.pallcare.info/> (accessed on 1 Feb 2014).

Regulations, legal duties, and financial support for patients

Regulations, legal duties, and financial support for patients

Introduction to regulations, legal duties, and financial support for patients

If you are reading this book cover to cover, you should, by now, have a pretty good idea of how to 'do palliative care' well. However, there a few rules you may need to know, most certainly if you are a medical student or doctor, although many nurses also need to know them. These rules cover:

+ prescribing controlled drugs (e.g. strong opioids);
+ prescribing drugs beyond licence;
+ how you can help patients to get financial support;
+ administrative duties after death.

Familiarity with these rules is important. Errors made in these areas can have a significant impact on patients or families and whilst some may be more of an inconvenience to you and others, all are a cause for embarrassment.

Prescribing controlled drugs (CDs)

The law regulates which CDs can be made, prescribed, supplied, and possessed, and by whom. Regulation is by the Misuse of Drugs Act 1971 and Misuse of Drugs Regulations 2001 and their amendments. The Misuse of Drugs Act 1971 prohibits certain activities in relation to 'controlled drugs', in particular their manufacture, supply, and possession. The penalties applicable to offences involving the different drugs are graded broadly according to the *harmfulness attributable to a drug when it is misused* and, for this purpose, the drugs are defined in the following three classes:

+ **Class A** includes strong opioids and class B substances when prepared for injection.
+ **Class B** includes oral amphetamines and codeine.
+ **Class C** includes most benzodiazepines.

The regulations lay down the conditions under which supply and possession can be carried out. The various controlled drugs are categorized into *schedules*, each specifying the requirements governing such activities as import, export, production, supply, possession, prescribing, and record keeping which apply to them.

◆ **Schedule 1** includes drugs which are not used medicinally. Possession and supply are prohibited, except in accordance with Home Office authority.

◆ **Schedule 2** includes drugs such as diamorphine and morphine, and are subject to the full controlled drug requirements relating to prescriptions, safe custody, and the need to keep registers.

◆ **Schedule 3** includes buprenorphine, midazolam, and temazepam. They are subject to some special prescription and safe custody requirements but records in registers do not need to be kept.

Schedule 4 and 5 drugs have less restriction. Table 7.1 shows the schedule for drugs which are used for symptom management in palliative care.

Prescriptions for Schedule 2 and 3 drugs are only valid for 28 days, and should not normally be for more than 30 days' supply. If a patient wishes to travel abroad with CDs, exceptions may be made but need to consider requirements for both leaving the United Kingdom and entering the foreign country. This is beyond the remit of this book but some guidance is given in the 'Resources' section at the end of the chapter.

It is very important to make yourself aware of local policies for issuing, collecting, transporting, and disposing of CDs. A person collecting or transporting Schedule 2 CDs (e.g. the patient's family member) must show their identification.

Table 7.1 Some CDs used in palliative care and their regulation schedule

Schedule 2	Schedule 3	Schedule 5
Morphine (except 10 mg in 5 ml oral liquid)	Midazolam	Low-strength oral morphine (10 mg in 5 ml)
Fentanyl, Alfentanil	Temazepam	
Diamorphine	Buprenorphine	
Oxycodone		
Hydromorphone		
Methadone		
Codeine injection		
Methylphenidate		

Note: Ketamine is Schedule 4 but, locally, may be treated as Schedule 2

Source: data from Misuse of Drugs Regulations 2001 (and subsequent amendments), available from <http://www.legislation.gov.uk/uksi/2001/3998/contents/made>, licenced under the Open Government Licence v2.0.

Writing the prescription

It is an offence to issue an incomplete CD prescription and, by law, a pharmacist cannot dispense it unless it is correctly written and will return it for re-writing if necessary. It's very important, therefore, to learn how to write a prescription for CDs correctly. This is shown in Figure 7.1. Common mistakes in prescription writing for CDs are shown in Box 7.1

All the usual prescription writing requirements apply, but you *must* also include the total quantity of whatever preparation(s) you are ordering in both *words and*

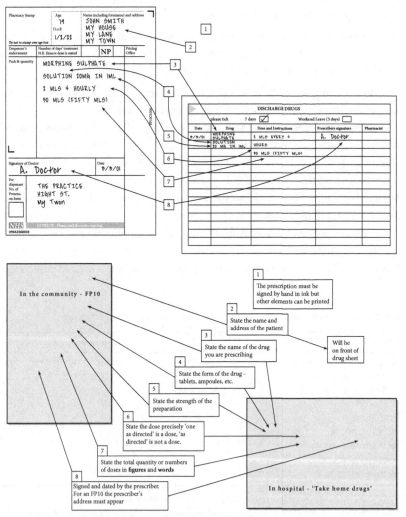

Figure 7.1 Example of an FP10 and 'TTO' (to take home) prescription for a controlled drug

Box 7.1 Common mistakes when writing prescriptions for controlled drugs

- Just writing 'PRN' or 'as directed', with no dose, is not legal.
- Don't forget to write the total quantity in both *words and figures*.
- *Sign in your own handwriting* and date your prescription.

 LEARNING EXERCISE

Ask to borrow a drug chart or photocopy an FP10 prescription and practise filling it in by writing a prescription for diamorphine 30 mg and cyclizine 30 mg by subcutaneous infusion over 24 hours. Check you've done it right by showing someone who knows (e.g. a pharmacist or doctor). **Tip**: don't forget to prescribe the water for injection as a diluent!

figures. Scripts must be written legibly in indelible ink. They can be typed or computer generated but must be hand signed. The information you must give is:

- The prescriber's address (and, as good practice, your GMC or NMC registration number)
- The patient's name and address
- The drug name
- The form of drug: sustained-release (SR) tablets, ampoules, oral liquid, or capsules
- The strength of the preparation(s): remember that more than one tablet/capsule strength may be required to make up the dose you want the patient to have
- The dose stated in appropriate units, e.g. mg, mg/ml, micrograms/hour
- The frequency to give the dose: for SR opioids this should be 12 hourly rather than BD. For opioids for breakthrough pain, this can be 'up to 2hrly'. You should look at the section 'The management of pain' in Chapter 5 to review your knowledge of this.

In addition to the prescription, which allows the pharmacist to dispense the drugs, nurses require clear written instructions ('authorization') from the responsible prescriber on how the drug should be administered. This is usually for drugs delivered by injection, either as intermittent doses or via a continuous infusion in a syringe driver. The authorization will not only need to include the drug, dose, route, and frequency but also the indication for the drug for example, 'give morphine 10 mg/24 hr sc for breathlessness'. If you also wanted to instruct the nurse to give morphine for pain, this would require a *separate, additional* authorization.

Remember to prescribe a diluent (e.g. water for injections or sodium chloride 0.9%)

Use of drugs beyond licence

Many drugs commonly used to provide excellent symptom management in palliative care are used in a way that does not comply with their licence. It may be that a licenced product is used for its licenced indication but in an unlicenced way (e.g. administration of a drug subcutaneously or via a feeding tube). Or it may be that a licenced product is used for an unlicenced indication (e.g. morphine for breathlessness). Mixing drugs in a syringe driver is another example of the use of drugs beyond their licence and is established practice in palliative care.

Such 'off-license' use is legitimate and allowed within established practice or where the risk is considered to be low. Greater caution is needed where the risk or benefit is more debatable or the risks are greater (e.g. intravenous route of administration).

The prescriber must act reasonably and responsibly, including:

◆ where possible or appropriate, gaining patient consent;

◆ recording the reasons for decisions in the patient record;

◆ discussing with other professionals. to avoid misunderstandings (e.g. wrong route errors).

Getting financial support for patients

For many patients and their families, sickness has devastating financial implications.

For example:

◆ they can no longer work;

◆ additional heating/electricity/water (perhaps extra laundry) costs;

◆ additional transport costs;

◆ possible contributions towards domiciliary care/support;

◆ costs for some aids and adaptations not provided by statutory agencies.

There are various ways patients can receive financial support:

◆ the State (e.g. Universal Credit, Employment and Support Allowance, Personal Independent Payments (previously Disability Living Allowance), Attendance Allowance, Carer's Allowance);

- private insurance schemes (only for those already paying in);
- charitable sources (Macmillan Cancer Support, local charities).

Each of these may require documentary evidence from a doctor or other health care professional. Someone else may handle much of this process but it is important for you to have an awareness of people's social situation. Many potential claimants miss out because no one thinks about their eligibility and the patient and family are unaware of what they are entitled to. Knowing the range of assistance available allows you to prompt thoughts, within the multi-disciplinary team, about financial support.

For patients who are terminally ill and have a short prognosis (i.e. who are not expected to live for more than 6 months), a doctor can sign a DS1500 form which enables patients to claim under 'special rules'. 'Special rules' is a fast track system that allows people, who are eligible, to receive payment quickly if they are claiming Personal Independent Payments or Attendance Allowance. This negates the need to wait for the usual qualifying period.

Also under 'special rules', if someone is making a claim for Employment and Support Allowance or Universal Credit, and a DS1500 form is appropriate (as required by the Department for Work and Pensions), they will be placed immediately into the Department's 'support group' category and awarded the highest rate of benefit. They will not be required to attend a medical assessment.

For more information about benefits see <https://www.gov.uk/browse/benefits/disability>

Death verification

Once a patient has died, the death will need to be confirmed. It might be hard to believe, but errors very occasionally happen when verifying death. The consequences of this do not need emphasizing! Also, delays in completing any of the formal after-death procedures can cause considerable distress and inconvenience to relatives. We need to get this right! Figure 7.2 illustrates the procedures around death verification. A death can be verified by a doctor and those paramedics and nurses who have undergone specific training and if local policies allow this. For an expected death, there is no hurry to verify it. Family can spend time with their loved one. However, they may want the support of a professional who can confirm what they think has happened.

Care after death

The nurses' and support workers' roles at the end of life extend beyond death to provide care for the deceased person and support to their family. The nurse and

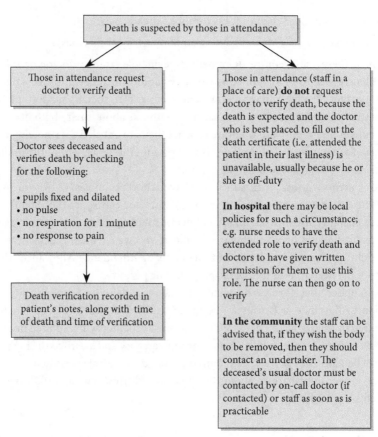

Figure 7.2 Process of death verification

support workers are also involved, sometimes with the family, in the preparation of the body. Care after death includes:

- honouring the spiritual and cultural wishes of the deceased person and their family;
- preparing the body for transfer to the mortuary or funeral director;
- offering the family and carers the opportunity to be involved, as much or as little, in the process and supporting them in this;
- ensuring the privacy and dignity of the deceased person is maintained;
- ensuring the health and safety of everyone who comes in contact with the body is protected;
- honouring the wish for organ or tissue donation;
- returning the deceased person's property to the relatives.

The personal care that a nurse may need to undertake for a deceased person can be daunting for some and it is important that student nurses and new health care assistants work alongside qualified and more experienced staff to gain experience in this and to be supported in their reactions to caring for a dead person. Elements of the care that may need to be provided are shown in Table 7.2.

Table 7.2 Care for a patient after death

Element of care	Details[1]
Working with family members and respecting cultural and religious requirements.	Some family members may wish to assist with the personal care, often in acknowledgement of individual wishes or religious or cultural requirements. Prepare them sensitively for changes to the body after death and be aware of manual handling and infection control issues. For some patients, the gender or religion of who is allowed to touch the deceased's body is very important and every effort should be made to comply with this value.
Equipment	When the death is not being referred to the coroner, remove mechanical aids such as syringe drivers, venous catheters, nasogastric tubes. Apply gauze and tape to syringe driver sites and document disposal of medication. Remove or spigot urinary catheters.
Positioning the body	Lay the deceased person on their back, adhering to manual handling policy; straighten their limbs (if possible) with their arms lying by their sides. Leave one pillow under the head as it supports alignment and helps the mouth stay closed. If it is not possible to lay the body flat due to a medical condition, then inform the mortuary staff or funeral director.
Eyes	Close the eyes by applying light pressure for 30 seconds. If this fails, then explain sensitively to the family/carers that the funeral director will resolve the issue. If corneal or eye donation is to take place, close the eyes with gauze (moistened with normal saline) to prevent them drying out.
Mouth	Clean the mouth to remove debris and secretions. Clean and replace dentures as soon as possible after death. If they cannot be replaced, send them with the body, in a clearly identified receptacle.

Table 7.2 (continued) Care for a patient after death

Element of care	Details[1]
Hair	Tidy the hair as soon as possible after death and arrange into the preferred style (if known) to guide the funeral director for final presentation.
Shaving	Usually, the funeral director will do this.
Leakage	Pads and pants can be used to absorb any leakage of fluid from the urethra, vagina, or rectum. Contain leakages from the oral cavity or tracheostomy sites by suctioning and positioning. Cover exuding wounds or unhealed surgical incisions with a clean, absorbent dressing and secure with an occlusive dressing. Leave stitches and clips intact. Cover stomas with a clean bag. Avoid waterproof, strongly adhesive tape as this can be difficult to remove at the funeral directors and can leave a permanent mark. If the body is leaking profusely, then take time to address the problem and inform the funeral director.
Dressing	Clean and dress the deceased person appropriately (use of shrouds is common practice in many acute hospitals). They should never go to the mortuary naked or be released naked to a funeral director. Be aware that soiling can occur.
Jewellery	Remove jewellery (apart from the wedding ring) in the presence of another member of staff, unless specifically requested by the family to do otherwise, and document this according to local policy. Be aware of religious ornaments that need to remain with the deceased. Secure any rings left on with minimal tape, documented according to local policy.
Identification	Clearly identify the deceased person with a name band on their wrist or ankle (avoid toe tags). As a minimum, this needs to identify their name, date of birth, address, ward (if a hospital in-patient), and, ideally, their NHS number. The person responsible for identification is the person who verifies the death.

Adapted from Wilson, J. and White, C., *Guidance for staff responsible for care after death*. National End of Life Care Programme and National Nurse Consultant Group (Palliative Care), © Crown Copyright 2011, available from <http://www.nhsiq.nhs.uk/media/2426968/care_after_death___guidance.pdf>, licenced under the Open Government Licence v.2.0.

Death certification

Once the death has occurred, then a death certificate needs to be issued. There is no hurry for the certificate to be written, so families need not be intruded upon, but only with this can the funeral directors and family then proceed with their funeral arrangements. The certificate also has a statuary function in that it is legal evidence of cause of death and provides epidemiological data. Only a doctor (or the coroner) can complete a death certificate.

The doctor who attended the deceased during their last illness is best placed to complete the death certificate, but he or she can only issue a death certificate if sure that:

- they know the cause of death;
- the patient had been seen by a doctor in the last 14 days;
- there are:
  - no suspicious circumstances
  - no evidence of violence
  - no links with an accident
  - no evidence of self-neglect or neglect by others (including medical care)
  - no links with an abortion
  - no suspicions of suicide
  - no suspicions of the death being linked to an industrial injury/disease
  - no suspicions that the death was related to medical treatment
  - no history of fractures
  - no evidence of a recent fall;
- the patient was not detained under the Mental Health Act;
- the patient was not recently held under police or prison custody;
- the patient was not in receipt of a war pension or industrial disability pension;
- the patient had not been operated on recently, or at least that full recovery from anaesthetic was achieved;
- the admission was not less than 24 hours.

If you have any doubt about whether to certify a death or not, then you can check the regulations, which can be found in the front of the death certificate book, or speak to the coroner or his/her officer. The coroner's teams are usually very helpful and may allow you to issue a certificate if the query is minor. They can be contacted via the local police station.

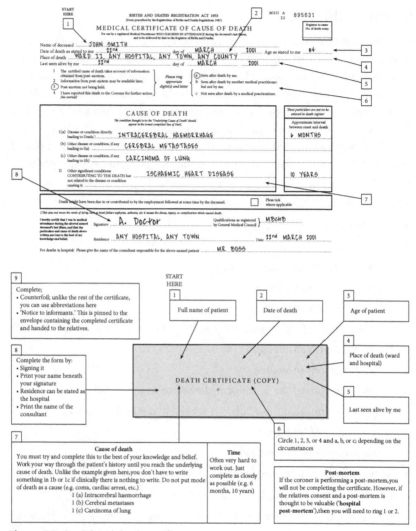

Figure 7.3 Completed death certificate

The rules around how to complete the death certificate are illustrated in Figure 7.3. Death certificates are taken by the family to the Register Office. The death must be registered within 5 days.

Cremation form

If the deceased is going to be cremated, then it is necessary for three doctors to examine the deceased and make an assessment of the cause of death. This is to make sure that there will be no mistakes necessitating any future need to examine the body. The form is in three parts. Cremation Form 4 is completed by the doctor who filled in the death certificate, and Cremation Form 5, by a second doctor who did not care for the patient in their last illness. Cremation Form 10 is completed by a crematorium medical referee.

Only a medical practitioner who treated the deceased during the last illness and who had seen him or her within 14 days of death should complete Cremation Form 4. Doctors completing Cremation Form 5 will need to speak to the patient's doctor and to someone who nursed the patient during their final illness. They may also need to speak with the relatives to be sure that there is nothing unexpected or worrying about the death from their perspective.

 SUMMARY BOX

There are administrative and legal duties required of doctors and nurses, and we need to be efficient at them. These include:

- prescribing strong opioids;
- prescribing drugs 'off licence';
- getting financial support for patients;
- verifying and certifying death;
- completing the cremation form.

 KEY POINTS

- There are rules which you must learn which affect the prescribing and administration of controlled drugs.
- Patients can access some financial support but you may need to sign a form to help them do this.
- Nurses, working sometimes with family members, may undertake particular tasks for a body after death.
- A death needs to be verified so that a body can be moved.
- A death needs to be certified by a doctor who knows the patient (or by the coroner).
- There are three parts to the usual cremation form which need to be completed by different doctors.

References

1. Wilson, J. and White, C. (2011) *Guidance for staff responsible for care after death.* National End of Life Care Programme and National Nurse Consultant Group (Palliative Care). Available at: <http://www.nhsiq.nhs.uk/media/2426968/care_after_death___guidance.pdf> (accessed 28th January 2014).

Resources

Using drugs beyond licence

British Pain Society. (2012) *Use of medicines outside of their UK marketing authorization in pain management and palliative medicine—information for patients.* This is a consensus document prepared on behalf of the British Pain Society in consultation with the Association for Palliative Medicine of Great Britain and Ireland. Available at: <http://www.britishpainsociety.org/book_useofmeds_patient.pdf> (accessed 28th January 2014).

British Pain Society and the Association for Palliative Medicine. (2005) *The use of drugs beyond licence in palliative care and pain management.* A position statement prepared on behalf of the Association for Palliative Medicine and the British Pain Society. Available at: <http://www.britishpainsociety.org/book_usingdrugs_main.pdf> (accessed 28th January 2014).

Medicines and Healthcare Products Regulatory Agency (MHRA). (2009) *Public consultation (MLX356); proposal for amendments to medicines legislation to allow mixing of medicines in palliative care.* Available at: <http://www.mhra.gov.uk/Publications/Consultations/Medicinesconsultations/MLXs/CON033523>

Taking controlled drugs abroad

Patients intending to travel abroad for more than 3 months, carrying any amount of drugs listed in Schedules 2, 3, or 4 Part I (CD Benz), will require a personal export/import licence. Further details can be obtained at <www.homeoffice.gov.uk/drugs/licensing/personal>

Applications must be supported by a covering letter from the prescriber and should give details of:

♦ the patient's name and address;
♦ the quantities of drugs to be carried;
♦ the strength and form in which the drugs will be dispensed;
♦ the country or countries of destination;
♦ the dates of travel to and from the United Kingdom.

Patients travelling for less than 3 months do not require a personal export/import licence for carrying controlled drugs, but are advised to carry a letter from the prescribing doctor.

Benefits and financial advice

Macmillan Cancer Support—

<http://www.macmillan.org.uk/Cancerinformation/Livingwithandaftercancer/Financialissues/Benefitsandfinancialhelp/Financialissues.aspx>

Citizens Advice—<http://www.adviceguide.org.uk>

Age UK—<http://ageuk.org.uk/money-matters/claiming-benefits/>

Chapter 8

Core competences
in palliative care

Chapter 8

Core competences in palliative care

How much palliative care do you need to learn?

One of the hardest things about learning is deciding what you need to know—how do you know what you don't know? For the student with their eyes on the next exam, the answer to this question is usually 'whatever the teacher decides' or, more honestly, 'what questions am I likely to be asked?' For the practicing health care professional, learning is less driven by exams and more by our professional ethic of wanting to do our best and to continue to develop our knowledge, skills, and attitude. Increasingly, though, revalidation is going to require us to demonstrate competence.

In 2009, to support the end of life care strategy, core competences were defined for health and social care workers.[1] We have used a tool, developed by a team in the East Midlands,[2] so that you can assess your areas of strength and weakness in the core competences.

Self-assessment as a measure of competence is not an entirely robust method, but it can be an excellent starting point. A further step would be for you to share your self-assessment with a senior colleague to gain their feedback on your performance.

How to use the self-assessment questionnaire

Go through the questionnaire in Table 8.1 and rate your assessment of your ability in a particular area by ticking the most appropriate box according to how you think you might do in an exam. Also write some reflection, in the comments box, about why you rate yourself at this level. It's useful to add a plan for your learning in this area. An example is given in Table 8.2.

You may find that there are large areas where you feel under-confident. Don't worry about this. This book will have many of the answers for you and you will pick up many other things in your training. You might need to look up things elsewhere; we've usually tried to give you guidance on this.

Table 8.1 A self-assessment questionnaire of the core competences in end of life care. Tick the relevant box for each question according to how you think you might do in an exam

Topic area	Imagine being assessed or asked a question about this in an exam. How would you do?					Comments
	Perform awfully ↔ Perform brilliantly					
	1	2	3	4	5	
Communication skills						
a. I feel confident to listen to and talk with a dying person about issues surrounding their death.						
b. I feel confident to listen to and talk with a relative of a dying person.						
c. I feel confident to communicate with a person with advancing illness who says to me 'I can see no meaning in life'.						
d. I feel competent to recognize a person's verbal/non-verbal cues.						
e. I feel confident that I can address a person's verbal/non-verbal cues.						
Assessment and care planning						
a. I understand the concept of holistic care.						
b. I use holistic assessment with people in my care.						
c. I feel able to recognize when a person is dying.						
d. I have a good understanding about the 'Gold Standards Framework'.						
e. My team use the 'Gold Standards Framework' for people in our care.						
f. I understand how to apply an individualized end of life care plan.						

Table 8.1 (continued) A self-assessment questionnaire of the core competences in end of life care. Tick the relevant box for each question according to how you think you might do in an exam

Topic area	Imagine being assessed or asked a question about this in an exam. How would you do?					Comments
	Perform awfully ↔ Perform brilliantly					
	1	2	3	4	5	
Symptom management, maintaining comfort and well-being						
a. I am confident about helping people with their pain.						
b. I am confident in using things other than drugs to help people to cope.						
c. I am confident in how to support a person in distress.						
d. I am comfortable discussing a person's anxiety about the dying process and what will happen.						
e. I am confident about helping people with the common symptoms they may experience at the end of life.						
Advance care planning						
a. I understand how 'advance care planning' enhances end of life care.						
b. When I am with a person with advancing disease who becomes unwell, I understand what their preferences are for the future.						
c. I recognize it is part of my role to find out what is known about a person's wishes should they lose capacity.						
d. If a person shares with me views about their future care, with permission, I would feel confident to discuss this with the wider care team.						

Table 8.1 (continued) A self-assessment questionnaire of the core competences in end of life care. Tick the relevant box for each question according to how you think you might do in an exam

Topic area	Imagine being assessed or asked a question about this in an exam. How would you do?					Comments
	Perform awfully ↔ Perform brilliantly					
	1	2	3	4	5	
Overarching values and knowledge						
a. I have thought about what is important to me in the meaning of my life.						
b. I recognize that my role is vital in delivering good end of life care.						
c. I feel my contribution to developing end of life care in my team is valued.						
d. I understand how society and culture influences attitudes to dying and death.						
e. I feel confident to be able to support a bereaved person.						

Reproduced with permission from Whittaker, B., Broadhurst, D., and Faull, C. *Evaluation toolkit: assessing outcomes of end of life learning events version 6*, East Midlands SHA, University of Nottingham, Copyright © 2013, available from <http://www.nottingham.ac.uk/research/groups/srcc/postgrad-course.aspx>

Table 8.2 Example of self-assessment to aid your learning.

Topic area	Imagine being assessed or asked a question about this in an exam. How would you do?					Comments
	Perform awfully ↔ Perform brilliantly					
	1	2	3	4	5	
I understand the concept of holistic care.			✓			*I know it's about the whole person but I always struggle to remember much about the spiritual aspects, especially as I am an atheist. I need to read and think about this a little more. Perhaps I might talk to a patient about it too.*

Table 8.3 Overall scoring of your assessment

Communication skills (C)		Assessment and care planning (A)		Symptom management, maintaining comfort and well-being (S)		Advance care planning (ACP)		Overarching values and knowledge (K)	
Question	Your score (out of 5)	Question	Your score (out of 5)	Question	Your score (out of 5)	Question	Your score (out of 5)	Question	Your score (out of 5)
a.		a.		a.		a.		a.	
b.		b.		b.		b.		b.	
c.		c.		c.		c.		c.	
d.		d.		d.		d.		d.	
e.		e.		e.				e.	
		f.							
Total (C) (out of 25)		Total (A) (out of 30)		Total (S) (out of 25)		Total (ACP) (out of 20)		Total (K) (out of 25)	
%		%		%		%		%	

To help you further, we have devised a scoring system which helps you identify broader areas of strengths such as being more able to do certain things or having a greater awareness of certain issues (albeit, perhaps still needing to know more). The scoring system is shown in Table 8.3 and how you might use the scores to consider you strengths and weaknesses is shown in Figures 8.1, 8.2, and 8.3.

For medical students and doctors in training, we have included a further questionnaire (Table 8.4) on physical symptoms, because competence in the management of these will be key for your role.

Scoring examples

Now, plot your total percentage scores for each of the areas of competence along the corresponding axes and join the marks together. From here, you can make some assessment of broad strengths or weaknesses. Examples of how this may look, with some accompanying comments, are given in Figures 8.1, 8.2, and 8.3.

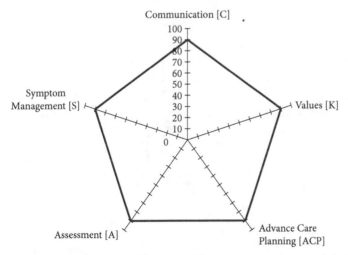

Figure 8.1 You are either over-confident or are about to apply to be a specialist in palliative care!

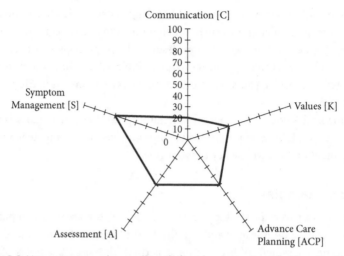

Figure 8.2 You seem strong in your knowledge about symptoms but less confident in communication with patients. It will be helpful to read Chapter 2 of this book and to undertake the learning exercises that are presented there.

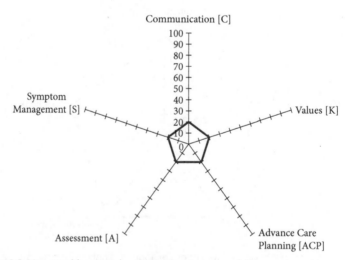

Figure 8.3 You are either grossly underestimating your abilities and need to prove to yourself you are better than this by doing some of the exercises in this book, or you need to speak to someone that can give you guidance!

Table 8.4 A self-assessment questionnaire for the management of common symptoms in palliative care

	Imagine being assessed or asked a question about this in an exam. How would you do?					Comments
	Perform awfully ↔ Perform brilliantly					
	1	**2**	**3**	**4**	**5**	
1. Understand that symptoms can be caused by the disease, treatment, or co-morbidity.						
2. Know how to take a pain history well.						
3. Diagnosis of different types of pain—pain can be categorized. Do you know any commonly used classifications?						
4. Appreciate that pain is not just a physical phenomenon, it is also social, psychological, and spiritual.						
5. An understanding of the array of drugs used for pain and the concept of opioid-sensitive pain.						
6. How to monitor the response to treatment.						
7. Sore mouth	For each of these symptoms, think of all the causes you can, how you would diagnose them, and the management options you know.					
8. Nausea and vomiting						
9. Constipation						
10. Diarrhoea						
11. Breathlessness						
12. Cough						
13. Anxiety, fear, and depression						
14. Acute confusional state (delirium)						
15. The indications for a syringe driver.						
16. An understanding of how to prescribe drugs which can be used in a syringe driver to manage common symptoms.						

SUMMARY BOX

It's crucial to know what is expected of you in your role in caring for patients and their families. The competences you require are in five domains: communication skills; assessment and care planning; symptom management, maintaining comfort and well-being; advance care planning; and reflection on your own, individuals', and society's thinking about death, dying, and bereavement. You should now have identified and thought about the gaps in your competences and how you might address them.

 KEY POINTS

♦ Core competences in end of life care have been defined for health and social care workers.

  Questionnaires can help you assess your level of competence

♦ The competences are in five domains:

  • communication skills,

  • assessment and care planning,

  • symptom management,

  • advance care planning,

  • reflection on your own, individuals', and society's thinking about death, dying, and bereavement.

♦ Self-assessment in each of the five domains is a starting point in helping you identify your strengths and weaknesses.

♦ You should make an action plan for your further development.

References

1. **Department for Health, Skills for Health, Skills for Care.** (2009) *Common core competences and principles for health and social care workers working with adults at the end of life.* London, Skills for Care. Available at: < http://www.skillsforcare.org.uk/Skills/End-of-life-care/End-of-life-care.aspx>

2. **Whittaker, B., Broadhurst, D., and Faull, C.** (2013) *Evaluation toolkit: assessing outcomes of end of life learning events version 6.* East Midlands SHA, University of Nottingham. Available at: <http://www.nottingham.ac.uk/research/groups/srcc/postgrad-course.aspx>

Further information about palliative care services and useful resources

Further information about palliative care services and useful resources

Who provides palliative care?

Palliative care is everyone's business and the palliative care principles discussed throughout this book can be offered by all health and social care professionals who are providing day-to-day care for patients and their carers in their own homes, hospitals, and in nursing or care homes. Sometimes, this may be referred to as generalist palliative care.

The National Council for Palliative Care[1] suggests that those providing generalist palliative day-to-day care should be able to:

- ◆ assess the care needs of each patient and their family in relation to their physical, psychological, social, and spiritual needs;
- ◆ meet those needs within the boundaries of their own knowledge, skills, and competence in palliative care (see Chapter 8);
- ◆ know when they need to seek advice from, or refer to, specialist palliative care services.

Specialist palliative care services

Palliative care in the United Kingdom, whatever the setting, is supported by an array of specialist multidisciplinary palliative care teams. The roles of specialist palliative care services are:

- ◆ to be a resource of specialist expertise, services, and sometimes equipment;
- ◆ as a specialist resource, to provide advice and support alongside the patient's usual doctor and nurse;
- ◆ to provide education;
- ◆ to train specialist practitioners;
- ◆ to undertake research.

If you are in any doubt about any aspect of palliative care, contact them. They are there to help you provide the best care for your patients. Get to know those that are local to you and how to make contact with them, and refer patients to the available services.

The components of a specialist palliative care service

Because of the historically unplanned provision of palliative care services (often provided by charitable organizations), the precise model of specialist palliative care services will differ between areas. In general, however, the elements available for you to find for your patients should be as follows.

The hospice

A hospice provides a service for people with advanced, progressive, life-threatening diseases. Hospices may be NHS funded or charitable. They may provide all or any of in-patient and out-patient care, day care, and care in the patient's home. This will vary from hospice to hospice; for instance, not all hospices will have in-patient beds. Most will also provide bereavement care of some form.

Home care

For many patients, a specialist nurse (sometimes called a Macmillan nurse; see the following section 'Palliative care nursing services') working in the community, alongside the primary health care team, is the only component of specialist palliative care they will need. If the specialist home care nurse works from a hospice or specialist palliative care unit, he or she will provide the contact point for the other components of the specialist service (e.g. medical advice, access to in-patient services).

Some home care teams will work 9 a.m. to 5 p.m., Monday through to Friday; other teams will provide a 24-hour service, 7 days a week.

Hospice at home

These teams aim to provide 24-hour care in the patient's own home in order to avoid unwanted admission and to help patients to return home from hospital in the very last days of life. They may sometimes also be part of Rapid Response Teams. Increasingly, patients needing intensive nursing care are being managed in their own homes.

In-patient care

In-patient care may be provided in designated palliative care beds, staffed by a specialist multidisciplinary team, in several different settings including specialist palliative care units or hospices and acute hospitals, community hospitals, or nursing homes. However, it is the team of professionals—their knowledge, skills, and philosophy of care—not the actual place of care that comprises specialist in-patient care (i.e. a hospice is not solely a building).

Patients may need admission for:

+ terminal care, when continued care at home is not possible and hospital or nursing home care is inappropriate because of the patient's and/or carer's specific needs;

+ short stays for complex symptom control;

+ respite care, in order to allow continued care in the community through adequate support of the carer;

+ rehabilitation for those with late-stage disease who require particular skills from staff, working together rapidly for realistic, achievable objectives outlined by the patient and the carer.

Day care

The day care unit can provide support for patients and respite to carers. It usually offers:

+ an environment of security, understanding, and mutual support, aiming to normalize the situation and provide control and choice in living with an advancing illness;

+ promotion of rehabilitation and help towards independence in activities of daily living;

+ support and therapy in the form of social activities, the relief of isolation and depression, and the general enhancement of well-being through, for example, chiropody, hair care, aromatherapy, and massage;

+ some nursing measures, including dressings and help with stoma care;

+ assessment, monitoring, advice, and intervention in symptom control;

+ access to medical advice;

+ discussion of diagnosis and prognosis.

Out-patient clinics

+ Clinics may be held in hospital specialist units/hospices or community health clinics.

+ Referral is usually made doctor to doctor.

+ Most provide general assessment, advice, intervention, and monitoring of physical and non-physical symptoms.

- Specific clinics may be provided by doctors and other health care professionals for:
  - the management of lymphoedema;
  - the management of breathlessness;
  - access to complementary therapies;
  - access to psychological support strategies (e.g. hypnosis, cognitive behavioural therapy);
  - nerve blocks and other interventional pain management techniques.

Hospital support teams

The hospital support team works mainly in an advisory capacity alongside other hospital professionals, e.g. in oncology, surgery, general medicine. The team requires a multiprofessional membership, similar to teams working in the community. Their role is:

- assessment of patient needs, e.g. symptom control, counselling, quality of life;
- specialist advice on symptom control and other needs;
- support, information, and advice to patients, families, informal carers;
- support, information, and advice to professional carers in hospital;
- education of professionals;
- promotion of continuity of care upon discharge of patient;
- research.

Bereavement support

The role of this service is to assess the need for support for carers and to offer this support in a carefully monitored and supervised way. Ideally, this work should begin before the death of the patient to prevent problems, particularly with those at risk of a difficult bereavement.

The service offered may comprise telephone contact, bereavement visiting, attendance at a bereavement group, bereavement counselling to individuals and families, and referral-on to other agencies. Some units may offer specific services for bereaved children.

Palliative care nursing services: who does what?

District nurse

District nurses play an important part in domiciliary palliative care. They provide hands-on nursing care, sometimes visiting the patients up to three times a day. The availability of night-time district nurses' services varies from area to area. They are contacted either via the GP surgery or their central base. The role of the district nurse is:

+ assessment of need;
+ general nursing care (e.g. dressings, pressure area care, bowel care);
+ emotional support to patients and their families;
+ health education and advice to patients and families;
+ often the key worker for patients and families in the community;
+ organizing equipment (e.g. mattresses, commodes, syringe drivers);
+ co-ordinating and accessing other services (GP, Marie Curie nurses, hospital nurses).

Marie Curie nurse

These nurses (of various grades) are organized and funded, in part, by the nationwide Marie Curie charity. They provide hands-on nursing care, staying with the patient for a number of hours, often overnight. This important service allows many patients to be managed at home, so avoiding inappropriate admissions for nursing care. They are contacted through a designated agency. The role of the Marie Curie nurse is:

+ 'hands-on' general nursing care;
+ emotional support to patients and their families;
+ emergency expertise by phone and in the patient's home in some areas where they are linked with urgent care, out-of-hours services.

Specialist palliative care nurse

Also known as Macmillan nurses or hospice home care nurses, these nurses will have usually added to their basic and post-registration education, a period of specific palliative care training. Some will be termed 'Macmillan nurses' in recognition of the charitable organization which funded their post initially. They usually work as part of a multiprofessional specialist team. The role of the specialist palliative care nurse is to:

+ assess the palliative care needs of patients;
+ bring specialist knowledge (e.g. symptom control, nursing care, ethical issues, decision making);
+ provide emotional support to patient, carers, and staff;
+ sometimes access hospice-based services (e.g. day care, additional aids, volunteers);

- sometimes provide bereavement follow-up;
- provide education.

SUMMARY BOX

Palliative care is the concern of every professional. However, sometimes you might need extra help and support. Knowing when you need help and where to get that help and information is important in ensuring you provide good care.

KEY POINTS

- Generalist palliative care is offered by all health and social care professionals.
- Specialist palliative care services are available to provide further care, support, and advice.
- There are a range of resources available to provide extra information and to support your learning.

References

1. The National Council for Palliative Care (NCPC). (2014) *Palliative Care Explained.* Available at: <http://www.ncpc.org.uk/palliative-care-explained> (accessed 4 February 2014).

Resources

The following addresses and websites provide useful information and resources for you and your patients on aspects of palliative care and on where to get more help. You may also find them useful to supplement your learning from this book.

Macmillan Cancer Support—cancer care and support charity

89 Albert Embankment, London SE1 7UQ, UK

Tel. 020 7840 7840

<http://www.macmillan.org.uk/>

Marie Curie Cancer Care—provide nursing care service to terminally ill people at home or in hospices

89 Albert Embankment, London SE1 7TP, UK

Tel. 020 7599 7729

<http://www.mariecurie.org.uk/>

National Council for Hospices and Specialist Palliative Care Services—umbrella charity for those working in palliative care in England, Wales, and Northern Ireland, working with the government, health and social care staff, and people with personal experience to improve end of life care for all

First Floor, 34–44 Britannia Street, London WC1X 9JG, UK

Tel. 020 7520 8299

<http://www.ncpc.org.uk/>

Scottish Partnership for Palliative Care—umbrella charity for those working in palliative care in Scotland, supporting and contributing to the development and strategic direction of palliative care in Scotland

1A Cambridge Street, Edinburgh EH1 2DY, UK

Tel. 0131 229 0538

<http://www.palliativecarescotland.org.uk/>

The Association for Palliative Medicine of Great Britain and Ireland—association for doctors who work or have an interest in palliative care

11, Westwood Road, Southampton SO17 1DL, UK

Tel. 01703 672888

<http://www.apmonline.org/>

Hospice UK—supports the work of hospices in the United Kingdom

34–44 Britannia Street, London, WC1X 9JG, UK

Tel. 020 7520 8200

<http://www.hospiceuk.org/#>

Together for Short Lives—a UK charity for children with life-threatening and life-limiting conditions

4th Floor, Bridge House, 48–52 Baldwin Street, Bristol BS1 1QB, UK

Tel. 0117 989 7820

<http://www.togetherforshortlives.org.uk/>

Cancer Help UK—provides reliable, easy to understand patient information from Cancer Research UK

<www.cancerresearchuk.org/cancer-help/>

Information about non-malignant advanced, progressive, life-threatening diseases

Alzheimer's Society

<http://www.alzheimers.org.uk/>

British Heart Foundation

British Kidney Patient Association

<http://www.britishkidney-pa.co.uk/>

British Liver Trust

British Lung Foundation

Motor Neurone Disease Association

<http://www.mndassociation.org/>

Multiple Sclerosis Society

<http://www.mssociety.org.uk/>

Parkinson's Disease Society

Terrence Higgins Trust (HIV and AIDS)

<http://www.tht.org.uk/>

Information about end of life care

Dying Matters—a coalition set up by the National Council for Palliative Care to promote public awareness of dying, death, and bereavement

<http://www.dyingmatters.org/>

e-ELCA (End of Life Care for All)—an e-learning project, commissioned by the Department of Health to enhance the training and education of health and social care staff involved in delivering end of life care

<http://www.e-lfh.org.uk/projects/end-of-life-care/>

End of Life (Social Care Institute for Excellence)—a resource for health and social care staff providing end of life care to adults

<http://www.scie.org.uk/adults/endoflifecare/index.asp#>

Gold Standards Framework

A systematic, evidence-based approach to optimizing the care for patients, nearing the end of life, delivered by generalist providers

<http://www.goldstandardsframework.org.uk/>

Leadership Alliance for the Care of Dying People (LACDP)—set up to lead and provide a focus for improving the care for dying people and their families

<http://www.england.nhs.uk/ourwork/qual-clin-lead/lac/>

National End of Life Care Intelligence Network—provides a national repository for sources of information on end of life care

<http://www.endoflifecare-intelligence.org.uk/>

National End of Life Care Programme—an NHS programme to improve end of life care for adults in England which closed on 31st March 2013 with the establishment of NHS Improving Quality (NHS IQ)

<http://webarchive.nationalarchives.gov.uk/20130718121128/http:/endoflifecare.nhs.uk>

Quality Standard for End of Life Care for Adults (National Institute for Health and Clinical Excellence; NICE)

<http://www.nice.org.uk/guidance/qs13>

Index